Praise for *Black Death at the Golden Gate*

"A medical detective story. . . . A mash-up of Erik Larson and Richard Preston. . . . [David K.] Randall is one of these writers who can take primary research—historical primary research—and just turn it into narrative."
　　　　　　　　—Tina Jordan, *New York Times Book Review* podcast

"A vivid, fast-paced and at times revolting history of the plague in San Francisco at the turn of the 20th century. [Randall] describes in chilling detail how the disease can overwhelm the human body. . . . [T]he book unfolds like a medical thriller. . . . With the latest upsurge in measles cases making the headlines, Mr. Randall's book is a timely reminder that public health challenges responsible for killing tens of millions of people world-wide are not confined to the past."　　　　　—Julia Flynn Siler, *Wall Street Journal*

"*Black Death at the Golden Gate* provides a fascinating glimpse into [a] forgotten chapter of American history. . . . Discrimination, bigotry, and greed are woven throughout this fast-paced, historical, non-fiction adventure. . . . This is a great read for anyone who enjoys history or medicine."—Jennifer Melville, *San Francisco Book Review*

"A fascinating, in-depth look at a little-known episode in American history. . . . The story of the bubonic plague outbreak serves as an excellent lead-in for Randall to examine the advances that created modern cities."　　　　　　　　　　　—*Shelf Awareness*

"This story of an epidemic that wasn't is a gripping historical mystery and a key cautionary tale for our own time."
　　　　　　　　　　　　　　　　　　　—*Booklist*

"A complex tale of medicine, politics, race, and public health. . . . [Randall] does good work in revealing the clamorous clash of public

and private interests surrounding the outbreak. . . . A tale that reso-
nates with the outbreak of measles, mumps, and other supposedly
contained epidemics today." —*Kirkus Reviews*

"David K. Randall has created a meticulously researched history
that unfolds like a thriller. I raced through this book in two days
(horribly, the span of time it took bubonic plague to fell a victim).
The unlikely heroes—bacteriologists and public health officers with
long, flowing beards—battle villains most vile: racism, rotten politics, disregard for science, and *Yersinia pestis*. *Black Death at the Golden
Gate* is both a page-turner and a cautionary tale: those villains still
lurk."—Mary Roach, *New York Times* best- selling author of *Grunt*

"A haunting detective tale packed with villains and heroes, *Black
Death at the Golden Gate* shows how bigotry and greed almost
brought a major U.S. city to ruin—and how science and courage
saved it. The events in this book may be a hundred years old, but its
message is as urgent as ever."
—Jason Fagone, author of the national bestseller
The Woman Who Smashed Codes

"David K. Randall is a spellbinding writer. He has turned a critical
chapter of medical history into a riveting tale that reads like a detective novel, chock-full of scandals and intrigue. . . . Read *Black Death
at the Golden Gate* because it's a page-turner, but more important,
read this book because the issues Randall spotlights resonate today."
—Randi Hutter Epstein, author of *Aroused*

BLACK DEATH
AT THE
GOLDEN GATE

BLACK DEATH

AT THE

GOLDEN GATE

THE RACE TO SAVE AMERICA FROM
THE BUBONIC PLAGUE

DAVID K. RANDALL

W. W. NORTON & COMPANY
Independent Publishers Since 1923

All rights reserved
Printed in the United States of America
First published as a Norton paperback 2020

For information about permission to reproduce selections from this book, write to
Permissions, W. W. Norton & Company, Inc., 500 Fifth Avenue, New York, NY 10110

For information about special discounts for bulk purchases, please contact
W. W. Norton Special Sales at specialsales@wwnorton.com or 800-233-4830

Manufacturing by Lake Book Manufacturing
Book design by Chris Welch
Production manager: Lauren Abbate

Library of Congress Cataloging-in-Publication Data

Names: Randall, David K., author.
Title: Black Death at the Golden Gate : the race to save America from the bubonic
plague / David K. Randall.
Description: First edition. | New York : W. W. Norton & Company, [2019] | Includes
bibliographical references and index.
Identifiers: LCCN 2018055377 | ISBN 9780393609455 (hardcover)
Subjects: LCSH: Plague—California—San Francisco—History—20th century.
Classification: LCC RC176.C2 R36 2019 | DDC 616.9/23200979461—dc23
LC record available at https://lccn.loc.gov/2018055377

ISBN 978-0-393-35815-5 pbk.

W. W. Norton & Company, Inc., 500 Fifth Avenue, New York, N.Y. 10110
www.wwnorton.com

W. W. Norton & Company Ltd., 15 Carlisle Street, London W1D 3BS

1 2 3 4 5 6 7 8 9 0

In memory of my father, Kenneth D. Randall,
the world's greatest storyteller

Such was the cruelty of heaven that between March and July upwards of a hundred thousand souls perished. What magnificent dwellings, what noble palaces were then depopulated! What families became extinct! What riches and vast possessions were left and no heir to inherit them! What numbers in the prime and giver of youth breakfasted in the morning with living friends and supped at night with their departed friends in the other world!

—Giovanni Boccaccio, *The Decameron*

CONTENTS

BLACK DEATH
AT THE
GOLDEN GATE

FIGHTING THE DEVIL
WITH FIRE

On the morning of December 8, 1899, Yuk Hoy, a forty-year-old bookkeeper, awoke in his bed to the flash of a high fever and a mysterious swelling in his thigh. Unable to do much more than mumble, he laid his head down and drifted in and out of sleep, largely ignored by the other men crammed into a windowless room of a two-story flophouse in Honolulu's overstuffed Chinatown. Having arrived just weeks before from his native China, Yuk Hoy had few friends in the bustling city, and his absence over the following days went unnoticed at the general store on Maunakea Street where he worked. Only his increasingly frantic cries alerted others to the misery of his existence. Woken by his wails, a man named Fong, who lived on the same floor, stumbled in darkness to find him trembling in a litter of straw, his body quivering, as Fong would later describe it, "like the branches of a tree in thunder and lightning gone crazy."

Fong lifted the man and made his way by moonlight along the unpaved streets of Chinatown to the office of Dr. Li Khai Fai on River Street one block away. Tall and fiery, Dr. Li was one of the few Chinese doctors trained in Western medicine that could be found in Hawaii, and he made little effort to hide his contempt for traditional Chinese healers whom he saw as clinging to a backward way of life. One of the few conciliations he made to what he regarded as superstition was to allow a friend to paint the table in the front room of his office deep red, the color of good luck. Other than that, his small office, only twelve feet across, was like that of any other Western-trained doctor, with a shelf full of books in English and a shiny brass spittoon by the front door.

Dr. Li was alone when Fong burst in and laid Yuk Hoy in front of him. The man was covered in feces and vomit and raved in apparent madness. Dr. Li struggled to hold his new patient still, all the while wondering how he was still alive. A finger to his wrist revealed a racing pulse, as if the body was facing an internal terror, while his forehead was so warm to the touch that Dr. Li fought the instinct to pull his hand away. When Yuk Hoy yelled, his screams sounded wet, as if emerging from below the sea. The man's skin, which days before had glimmered in the balmy Hawaiian sun, was pocked with black spots and open red sores, leaving the line between bodily tissue and the outside world an unsettled question. The lymph nodes in his thigh were so swollen that it looked as if his leg had been pumped full of air and was at risk of floating away. A mixture of blood and foam began leaking out of his mouth, a sign of ruptured blood vessels, and he soon fell into a coma from which Dr. Li knew he would never recover.

The doctor shuddered, wishing that what he saw before him was not real. He was one of only a handful of people then living in Hawaii who had seen the full power of the disease killing the man in front of him, and his knowledge had come at great personal cost. At the age of nine he had watched as his father, whose conversion to Christianity had led others in their village in southern China to call him a "running dog of the white devils," came under attack by a mob that stoned him to death in the street. His mother fled with her four children to Hong Kong, and at the age of sixteen Li enrolled at the Canton Medical School, a school of Western medicine founded by an American doctor from Ohio. There he met his future wife,

Dr. Kong Tai Heong, who in time would be at his side to witness death on a scale neither could have imagined.

Short where he was tall, reserved where he was loud, Dr. Kong was the physical opposite of her husband, yet she was widely seen as his intellectual superior. Left in a basket on the steps of a Lutheran mission in Hong Kong as an infant with nothing more than a pin bearing her name, she had grown up helping German nuns care for other children in her orphanage. They, in turn, helped her apply to the Canton Medical School. There she was known as the most brilliant student in her class, and, with Li, spent her off hours tending to victims of the epidemic ravaging Hong Kong that left hospitals reporting a 95 percent death rate. The pair graduated from medical school one June morning and were married in a Lutheran chapel the same afternoon. The following day they boarded a steamship headed to Hawaii, drawn by its promise of paradise after the hell they had seen. They entered Honolulu weeks later to the sound of cannon blasts, each one marking the island's celebration of the American Independence Day.

There was no doubt in Li's mind that the disease that he had prayed would never follow him had now come ashore. Since arriving in Honolulu, he had built up his practice ministering to poor Chinese immigrants who were suspicious of the small but powerful group of white merchants and missionaries who, two years earlier, had overthrown Hawaii's monarchy in hopes of American annexation. Any cooperation with the new government would be seen as a betrayal and put him at risk of meeting the same fate as his father. Despite that danger and the late hour, Dr. Li summoned Dr. George Herbert, an English physician who worked for the Board of Health. By the time he arrived, Yuk Hoy was dead. Dr. Herbert called in two other colleagues, and, with Dr. Li, prepared the examining table to conduct an autopsy in the small hours of the night.

By the flickering light of kerosene lanterns, the team of white doctors stood shoulder to shoulder and watched as Dr. Li opened the body and peeled back its skin to reveal signs of extensive internal hemorrhaging. Dr. Li pointed to the black marks on the arms, the dried blood in the mouth, and the swollen lymph nodes in the armpits, neck and groin. The procedure finished, Dr. Li told the men in front of him in his halting English that the man's symptoms perfectly matched those he had seen among the dead of Hong Kong. His voice echoed in the silent room. Dr. Walter Hoffman, a young German doctor just four months into his job as Honolulu's first bacteriologist, stepped forward to take a sample of tissue from the glands of the dead man. His laboratory across town was the only place on the island that could confirm what every doctor assembled that night now believed: for the first time in history, bubonic plague had reached Hawaii, bringing with it the capacity to kill everyone they loved in a matter of days.

On the eve of the modern era, one of the most feared diseases in human history returned without warning and unleashed death on a scale not seen in centuries. Bubonic plague appeared in the rural province of Yunnan in south central China in the late 1870s, where it festered for nearly two decades before making its way across the globe. By 1893 it had reached the city of Canton, where, in the words of one observer, it killed thousands of people "like plum blossoms in a late frost." From there, the disease traveled along the Pearl River to Hong Kong, and then on board steamships to the wider world. In China, some ten million people died within a span of five years; by the end of 1910, another five million would perish as plague emerged in India, Australia, Scotland, and North Africa, sparking fears that the Black Death—a fourteenth-century worldwide outbreak of plague that in some areas killed 60 percent of the population—had returned.

The disease seemed to arrive with no cause and overwhelm the body with no cure. In 1894, a tiny, rod-shaped bacterium known as *Yersinia pestis* was identified as the source of plague, but beyond that little else—how the disease spread, who was most likely to contract it, or whether any medicines could dent its progress—was known. Doctors engulfed in the first clash between the ancient disease and modern medicine were left to experiment for themselves, knowing all the while that millions of lives hung in the balance. Coming at a time when public health officials were widely distrusted—during the smallpox epidemic of 1894–95 in Milwaukee, Polish women armed with baseball bats and butcher knives patrolled the streets ready to combat health inspectors they feared were using disease as a cover to confiscate their homes and belongings—the fight against plague would prove to be a battle over the legitimacy of science, laying the foundation for a century of public health improvements that extended the life span of the average American by nearly thirty years.

With so much about the disease a mystery, its name alone was spoken with dread. Though few living at the time had any firsthand experience with plague prior to its reappearance, the trail of dead that it had once left in its wake made it seem like nothing short of divine wrath. A 1665 outbreak of plague in London sparked terror so great "that the courage of the people appointed to carry away the dead began to fail them; nay, several of them died, although they had the distemper before, and were recovered; and some of them dropped down when they had been carrying the bodies even at the pit side, and just ready to throw them in; and this confusion was greater in the city, because they had flattered themselves with hopes of escaping and thought the bitterness of death was past," wrote Daniel Defoe in *Journal of the Plague Year*, fifty-seven years after the epidemic.

Prejudice often filled in the blanks. Puzzled by the fact that few upper-class foreigners living in colonial compounds in Hong Kong and India caught the disease even as thousands around them succumbed, some public health officials drew the pseudoscientific conclusion that those with European ancestry had somehow developed immunity to plague and pointed to their survival as proof of racial superiority. In 1897, the powers of Europe, nervous at the thought of allowing someone bearing the disease across their borders, agreed to impose travel restrictions on goods and people that codified this theory into law, allowing upper-class whites free passage from plague-stricken areas while denying entry to everyone else.

With its arrival in Chinatown, the path of plague in Honolulu seemed to confirm what many white Hawaiians already suspected. On the night of Yuk Hoy's death, another Chinese bookkeeper was found dead with the same symptoms just blocks away. Five additional victims were discovered over the next four days, all of them Chinese men except for one twenty-four-year-old man who had days before arrived from the Gilbert Islands, some two thousand miles away. The Board of Health ordered a five-day quarantine of Chinatown, trapping an estimated ten thousand men and women in the space of eight city blocks. Armed guards stood with fixed bayonets at the edge of the district, intent on keeping anyone infected with the disease from spreading it beyond its borders. A mob soon gathered outside the office of Dr. Li, the man they now blamed for their confinement. The doctor jumped on his bicycle and raced away, barely escaping with his life. As rumors of an imminent riot bubbled through the city, the Board of Health counted down the days until it could lift the quarantine, hoping that their nightmare would soon end.

On the day that the barriers were set to come down, a German teenager named Ethel Johnson developed a suspiciously high fever. The modest Johnson home was on Iwelei Road, a street just outside the quarantine zone that bent from the edge of Chinatown toward the harbor. Wagons filled with human waste, collected from the toilets of the district, were a common sight traveling past the house en route to a seaside dump. A team of doctors sent to the girl's home found suspicious lumps in her armpits and groin, leaving them no choice but to identify her as a possible case of plague. A phalanx of soldiers formed a barrier around the Johnson home, blocking anyone from entering or leaving the residence, despite the protests of a physician at the Board of Health who found it an insult to group the girl together with "Hawaiians, Japanese and Chinese, an act which would defile the dignity of [her] whiteness, the people who control and rule this archipelago."

Ethel Johnson died five days later. Other deaths followed in rapid succession, like dominos spreading across a table. On Christmas Eve, a twenty-seven-year-old Chinese laborer by the name of Ah Fong fell dead in a vegetable garden; on Christmas Day, the body of a twenty-four-year-old Chinese man named Chong Mon Dow was found in a shack, placed there by one of the sixteen other men who shared a room with him in Chinatown. The next day, doctors at the Wai Wah Yee Yuen hospital in Chinatown discovered the body of a twenty-five-year-old man dumped in the street outside its gate, teeming with plague.

With the quarantine ineffectual, the Board of Health panicked, consumed by the prospect of the islands becoming overwhelmed by a disease that seemed to have no cure. The men then turned to what even they agreed was a solution that would have seemed crazy six weeks before: fire. No science could point to its efficacy, and no city had ever tried it before, but the prospect of burning the disease away satisfied some deep urge.

Nathaniel Emerson, the eldest member of the board, stood at a podium before the group of men who effectively ruled all of Hawaii. The son of missionaries from New England, he was one of the few white adults who had been born on the islands and had sailed east to attend Williams College in his parents' native Massachusetts. While he was there, the Civil War broke out, and he enlisted in defense of a nation to which his home did not technically belong. Scars from Confederate artillery shrapnel that wounded him during the Battle of Gettysburg still traced his body. He returned to the islands years later, after earning a medical degree at Harvard and then working as a private physician in Manhattan. He brought with him a thoroughly Yankee sensibility, which often seemed out of place in a land of sugarcane and pineapple. At the age of sixty, he no longer feared the social consequences of his actions and prided himself on his independence.

"I am willing to go right ahead and take all the responsibility and burn anything and do anything that is necessary," he told the men seated before him. One by one, his colleagues agreed. They would burn every building suspected of harboring plague to the ground immediately, regardless of the owner's wishes, praying that fire could do what medicine so far could not. On the morning of Saturday, December 31, local firemen ignited a pair of two-story buildings where a man named Ah Kau had been found dead of plague a few days before. The buildings were home to eighty-five Chinese, Japanese and Hawaiians, who were all taken to a make-shift quarantine station that resembled a prison. English-language newspapers cheered the new policy, with the *Commercial Advertiser* calling it "fighting the devil with fire."

As the flames overwhelmed the buildings, black smoke rose high into the deep blue skies. Fire was the city's last hope, and no one knew if it would work. No New Year's Eve celebrations were held in Honolulu that evening, the final night of the nineteenth century. The only sound in the deserted city's streets was that of a Portuguese band, playing the wailing notes of a funeral dirge.

CHAPTER I

ACROSS THE SEA

His banishment now felt complete.

Six weeks earlier, Joseph Kinyoun had been heading into middle age ensconced in a bubble of his own brilliance. Widely seen as one of the most accomplished scientists in the United States at the age of thirty-nine, he was still young enough to expect that his achievements were a prelude to greatness. He spent his days in a laboratory built to his specifications, which was without question the finest in North America, located so close to the Capitol building that the view from his fourth-story window consisted of little more than its blinding white rotunda. At night, he went with his wife, Lizzie, to the finest restaurants in Washington, where he spent hours in conversation with sitting senators, his reputation as one of the youngest to ever climb the ranks of the Marine Hospital Service an entryway to the social heights of a city that still felt Southern a generation after the Civil War. He expected nothing less than for his life to continue along the same upward trajectory that it always had.

One order from Surgeon General Walter Wyman, the only man who outranked him in the Marine Hospital Service—the precursor to the modern U.S. Public Health Service—changed all that. Kinyoun had worked with Wyman for more than a decade, fulfilling his orders without question and offering advice when asked. Wyman marveled at the laboratory skills of Kinyoun, which he knew he would never be able to match, yet was unable to temper his envy as he watched Kinyoun's star outshine his own. At the age of fifty-one, Wyman was a lifelong bachelor who over his nine years heading the Marine Hospital Service had set rules governing every aspect of the job, down to the proper wording of memos and the correct angle at which the dress uniform's ceremonial sword should hang from an officer's hip. Suspicious of any threat to his control, Wyman developed a habit of issuing sudden transfer orders to any officer who gained public acclaim, leaving one longtime Service member to say, "He found out where you didn't want to go—and he sent you there."

Wyman's resentment of Kinyoun built slowly over several years, and then cascaded down shortly after the *Journal of the American Medical Association*—a publication read by every doctor in the country and by the Marine Hospital Service officers posted at more than twenty ports overseas—published an issue in which it repeatedly referred to Kinyoun as the true Surgeon General and called Wyman unfit for his job. Though Kinyoun had never outwardly encouraged the attention, Wyman drew up a letter in early May of 1899 notifying him that he was to immediately report to a new station on the other side of the country. For the rest of his life, Wyman would take pains to avoid mentioning Kinyoun by name.

A hastily arranged farewell dinner was held in Kinyoun's honor in an upstairs ballroom at Rauscher's, a French restaurant then at the top of Washington's social hierarchy. Fifty of the most lauded doctors in the country—a group that included George Sternberg, the sitting U.S. Army Surgeon General, and Z. T. Sowers, whose work championing the accurate labeling of drugs would lead to the creation of the Food and Drug Administration—listened while Professor George M. Kobe, soon to be dean of the Georgetown Medical School, reminded the group of Kinyoun's genius. "No member of his corps has contributed more to the reputation of the Marine Hospital Service and helped to place it upon a higher scientific plane than Dr Kinyoun," he said. In an understated dig at Wyman, who did not attend the ceremony, he added, "It seems a pity, therefore, that this modest, unassuming scientist should be divorced from a laboratory which has already accomplished so much and promised still more for the future usefulness of this branch of the public service."

Kobe revealed to the men around him that Kinyoun had received the tempting offer of a full professorship at Rush Medical College in Chicago, yet turned it down because he felt that his first duty was to the public welfare of his country. "Men of this type are rare in the world, especially in these days of struggle for wealth and fame, when the accelerated speed of the race has quickened the pulse, stimulated the nerves and fired the ambition of men, until they overleap all limits of propriety," he said. "It is not so with our honored guest, for he evidently belongs to the descendants of that noble band of patriots, ready to defend a principle with their lives, their fortune and their sacred honor."

Before the month was over, Kinyoun, along with his pregnant wife and three young children, climbed aboard a train bound for San Francisco and a coast they had never before seen. They reached California twelve days later, following long stops in Denver and Salt Lake City to allow Lizzie to get some rest. Even with the unexpected delay, their new quarters at the Marine Hospital station in San Francisco were not ready when they arrived. The city itself seemed unwilling to greet them, consumed by a dense fog and chilly wind that felt like a closed door. A small earthquake that jolted the city the next day only confirmed the sense that California wanted nothing to do with them.

The Kinyoun family spent several days at the enormous Palace Hotel, which stretched across an entire city block at the corner of Market and Montgomery streets downtown and offered a level of elegance that prompted the steel magnate Andrew Carnegie to once proclaim, "There is no hotel building in the world greater than this." Kinyoun, however, found the pageantry of the place an affront to his natural frugality, and shepherded his family toward the docks as soon as he received word that their new home was ready. The family boarded a private ferry for the thirty-minute trip to Angel Island, a hilly, star-shaped outpost that would be their home for the foreseeable future. There, on the largest island in the San Francisco Bay, Kinyoun took charge of the thirty-two-building complex that made up the most extensive quarantine station in the country, and which was responsible for inspecting all passengers and goods arriving through the Golden Gate.

Before leaving Washington, Kinyoun had extracted a promise from Wyman that he would be able to continue his laboratory research in California as time permitted. Upon arrival, however, he realized that would be impossible. The wharf where the ferryboat docked—and, indeed, the island's only connection to the outside world—was so close to tumbling down that Kinyoun wondered if it was even possible to land. The station itself, meanwhile, was running dangerously short of water, holding so little reserve supplies that a malfunction of one of the hundreds of kerosene lamps required in the absence of electric light threatened to burn down the entire wooden complex. Microscopes and other laboratory equipment sat untouched in dirt-covered boxes. No working telephone or telegraph connected the island to the mainland, and the boats quarantine officers used to meet incoming vessels were so slow and top-heavy that they risked injury every time they went on patrol.

Every ship that appeared out of the fog stitched through the Golden Gate made the situation worse. Dozens of passengers on board a steamship from Hawaii might be discharged on the island at the same time as a crew of merchant sailors from Japan and the members of a Russian whaling party returning from Alaska, the jumble of languages and smells leaving Kinyoun all the more unmoored. The world arrived at his doorstep by the hour, united only by the fact that no one wanted to spend another minute waiting for inspections before they were allowed clear passage on to San Francisco. If he did need to treat a sick passenger, he had little to offer. The main hospital on the island was in shambles, with patients infected with communicable diseases sharing small rooms with men and women there for quarantine, a layout that practically begged for illness to spread. Every night, Kinyoun retreated to a small wooden barrack that served as his new home, where a cold wind from the bay seeped through the walls and left him perpetually worried that his children were about to fall sick. Worse yet, he did not know what else lay in store for him. Simply making a full tour of the island was rendered nearly impossible after a surprise summer rain washed the dirt roads away.

Adding to Kinyoun's humiliation, he soon discovered that dozens of acres of the otherwise pristine and uninhabited island were covered in garbage, the only remaining evidence of the thousands of troops who had passed through quarantine after returning from the Philippines at the conclusion of the Spanish American War. The kind of scientific progress that had propelled his rise was now replaced by the opportunity to clean up trash, all the while literally marooned on an island on the other side of the continent from everyone and everything he considered important. "I heard a joke, which I consider quite a good one, on me a few days ago, and that was that rumor had reached San Francisco that I had been sent here by the Surgeon General to be buried," Kinyoun wrote to a friend in Washington as he began work on bringing the station up to his standards. "Don't you think that I have been rather a lively corpse, if that was the reason?"

In many ways, Kinyoun's levity masked a rawness that had not diminished with age. With his thinning brown hair, stocky body and gold wire-rim glasses perched above a trim dark beard, Kinyoun looked more the part of a member of the Eastern elite than his life history would suggest. His unquestioning self-confidence had launched him from the humblest beginnings and now sustained him as he faced the indignity of his new surroundings.

It was not the first time that his personality had provoked scorn. At a time when there were few men or women in America that he considered his intellectual equals, he was accustomed to being right, and, like many researchers whose brilliance is most apparent in the laboratory, he lacked the social intelligence to smooth over disagreements. As a result, he often tangled even with those who liked him, flashing a stubbornness that frequently threatened to push his objectives further out of view. The sudden posting to San Francisco, which he considered a public rebuke by Wyman, only brought the darker aspects of his personality to the surface.

His willfulness had been fostered by a childhood marked by upheaval. He was born on the eve of the Civil War in the remote hill country of East Bend, North Carolina, into a wealthy family that owned slaves. When Joseph was five months old, his father, John, left his small medical practice to join the Confederate Army, in whose service he fought in thirteen successive battles before resigning as a captain to work as a surgeon at a hospital in the rebel capital of Richmond, Virginia. He was among the thousands of men who surrendered to General Sherman in Durham, North Carolina, immediately following Lincoln's assassination, and soon returned to East Bend, only to discover that his home had been burned down and nearly all of his farmland destroyed. After a brief stint in Texas, John Kinyoun resettled his family in the frontier town of Oak Township, Missouri, where he made his living splitting railroad ties for about a dollar a day.

The small town, nestled near the Kansas border, had been settled mostly by refugees from Southern states, and soon became a lawless place of vigilante justice among men who refused to let the Civil War die. There, Joseph Kinyoun spent his childhood in a small log cabin, where he devoured Greek and Roman classics and taught himself French, German and Spanish as an escape from the violence all around him. At the age of sixteen he began to study medicine under his father's tutelage, a practice common at a time when most would-be physicians learned their craft in informal apprenticeships like blacksmiths. Under his father's guidance, he learned how to diagnose common ailments, how to clean a wound and, most importantly, how to be quick with a knife when anesthesia was an indulgence. By the age of twenty-one, he was ready to move to New York City to study at Bellevue Hospital, one of the few places in the country that could offer formal research experience at a time when most hospitals were sparse, primitive wards.

In New York, Kinyoun took the first steps in his transformation from country doctor into one of the giants of the burgeoning era of medicine in which laboratory skills would prove to be more consequential than bedside manner. He took courses in microbiology, analytical chemistry and infectious diseases, becoming one of the first Americans to harness the power of the microscope to target bacteria, which had only recently been identified as the true cause of disease. He graduated from Bellevue in the spring of 1882 and returned home to practice medicine in Missouri.

The loss of his first patient that winter—a young girl suffering from diphtheria, among the deadliest of childhood diseases—left him so depressed that he nearly quit the field. He consoled himself by buying a microscope, which was then considered more a toy for the idle rich than a crucial tool for medicine, and immersed himself in the study of agricultural diseases like anthrax and chicken cholera, all the while supporting himself by tending to women in labor for the price of ten dollars per delivery. Within three years he was married to Susan Elizabeth Perry, the daughter of a prominent Missouri family who asked that everyone call her Lizzie, and ready to break out of a comfortable rural existence that offered few avenues for intellectual adventure.

He returned to New York in 1885 as a newly married man to study as one of the first students at a bacteriological research laboratory at Bellevue funded by Andrew Carnegie. It soon became clear that his timing could not have been better. "The word 'bacteriology' had appeared before 1886 but the subject had no existence anywhere much before that time," noted William Thompson Sedgwick, one of the founders of the Harvard School of Public Health, in an early history of the field. A little more than two hundred years earlier, a Dutch tradesman and amateur scientist by the name of Anton van Leeuwenhoek had been the first to identify bacteria after experimenting with samples of lake water under an early microscope. Yet it would take more than a century for his discovery to find its application within medicine. With a previously unseen world now in view, the concept of disease began to morph from the medieval theory of miasma—the idea that so-called "bad air" spread infection—to pinpointing the exact bacilli that caused illness.

The new field of bacteriology focused more on cells than on the individual attributes of patients, and concerned itself chiefly with understanding how bacteria functioned in order to defeat it. Established doctors at the time considered this approach cold and unseemly, divorced from all the elements of humanity that made medicine feel so visceral, and remained unconvinced that laboratory work could offer anything that would alleviate a patient's suffering. Those objections became moot after early bacteriologists discovered how to grow pure colonies of bacteria in a lab setting and develop weakened strains of disease as a form of vaccine, opening a new era in which science could target the specific cause of a deadly illness in hopes of eliminating its spread. The results—coming at a time in which unsanitary medical care and overcrowding doomed one in five children born in New York City to die before their first birthday, and in which only three out of four adults lived past the age of thirty—seemed otherworldly, as if Prometheus had returned and stolen another secret of the gods.

As the Carnegie Laboratory's first bacteriology student, Kinyoun focused his research on cholera, an often fatal disease of the small intestine then uncommon in the United States, contracted from drinking infected water. He joined the Marine Hospital Service the following year, drawn by the chance to help fight disease on a scale he could scarcely imagine. With the advent of steamships and railroads, never before had the world seemed so small, and the Service, with its worldwide reach, offered the opportunity to save millions of lives. "The nations of the earth are more nearly related than ever before in the world's history," Surgeon General Wyman noted in a speech during Kinyoun's first years in the Service. "All the world has become one neighborhood, as far as relates to distances. In no manner has this been better shown than in the warfare against contagion . . . [which is] bringing the nations together as one family in the struggle against these foes of mankind."

Kinyoun soon set up the nation's first federal bacteriology laboratory in a quarantine station in Staten Island. There, in a small ground-floor room lined with bookshelves nearly touching the ceiling, he spent nearly all his waking hours peering into microscopes, hoping to isolate disease-carrying bacteria. One month into his research, an Italian ship arrived in New York harbor reporting the suspicious deaths of eight passengers en route. With the cause of death vague and the city at risk of introduction of a deadly disease, Kinyoun obtained tissue samples from the dead. Within a few days, he was able to isolate the bacilli that caused cholera, making him the first person in the Western Hemisphere whose laboratory work resulted in the positive identification of the disease. His research skills allowed public health officials to take swift steps to prevent cholera from establishing a foothold in New York, and turned him into a minor hero inside the rapidly professionalizing circles of American medicine.

His glory was soon cut short by the death of his three-year-old daughter, Bettie, who contracted diphtheria and died despite Kinyoun's frantic efforts to save her. Unable to go on working as before, he stepped down from his post as the head of the National Hygienic Laboratory and traveled to Europe, where he studied alongside pioneers in the field such as Louis Pasteur in Paris and Robert Koch in Berlin. With formal medical training still a rarity in the United States, Europe was at the time the center of research and drew countless ambitious young men and women from across the globe with its promise of discovery.

It was there, he would later say, that he fully understood that he stood at the start of a "new epoch." He watched as researchers tested the first antitoxin to counteract diphtheria, all the while imagining Bettie's face on every child injected with the experimental solution. He could only stand in wonder as dying children began to recover as if by magic. The effect was "so astounding that at first one is almost compelled to ask one's self, 'is this possible?'" Kinyoun wrote. Unable to trust what he was seeing, he conducted a study of hospital wards and laboratories to try to disprove what seemed like a miracle. Only then was he satisfied enough to trust it, writing a report back to Washington in which he admitted, "I have tried hard to find fault, to pick flaw in the statistics, but have signally failed. The work must stand for itself."

He returned to the States with a renewed sense that all infectious disease could be prevented by laboratory research. By his posting to San Francisco in early June of 1899, Kinyoun had invented some of the world's first disinfecting machines, prepared and tested the first smallpox serum in humans, developed new methods to fumigate railcars in order to prevent the spread of germs, and been called upon by Congress to investigate and remedy the poor ventilation of the House chambers. Yet as he spent the long afternoons of his first summer in the San Francisco Bay trying to get the Angel Island station in order, all that seemed nothing more than stories from a different person's life.

His time was engulfed by the endless work of inspecting passengers and cargo, and any spare moment went to tackling one of the many projects that nagged at him. All the while, he forced himself to don the Service's newest uniform, personally designed by Wyman, that featured gold epaulettes which left him feeling ridiculous and made it impossible to carry his youngest son, John, without the boy scratching his nose. "I do wish that they would have left the uniform alone," he complained in a letter to a friend. "I sincerely hope that the man who advocated these latest changes is supremely happy and contented. I have not found anyone so far with whom I have talked that gladly welcomes the additions."

Though it sat right across the bay, San Francisco remained a mystery to him. His work was so demanding that he only knew the city from the glimpses he got through the fog, finding himself so tired that he would find time to venture into the city at night only four times during his first year in California. The few hours he did spend in the city, however, left him cold, unable to reconcile what he saw as its blinding pursuit of profit with what he thought of as the higher purpose of life. Doctors and politicians who should have been his natural friends and allies went unmet, making his island home feel even more solitary. Physicians working at the Marine Hospital Service station in the Presidio district, meanwhile, remained indifferent to his attempts at friendship, the result of a lingering professional jealousy that the quarantine station at Angel Island did not fall under their jurisdiction. "The medical profession of San Francisco I know but little about," Kinyoun admitted in a letter to a friend back home. "When evening came, we were all so tired that, farmer like, we went to bed with the chickens."

On nights when he could not sleep, Kinyoun listened to the faint sounds of the city drifting across the bay. His thoughts often returned to his unused laboratory equipment, whose gathering dust sometimes seemed as if it had been placed there by Wyman himself to mock him. The field of bacteriology was advancing so rapidly that Kinyoun feared that he would be left behind, and felt all the dreams that he had for himself dissolving away. The posting to Angel Island threatened "to make such a break in my scientific work that it will be impossible for me to ever catch up again," he admitted in a letter to a friend.

His only hope was that Wyman would relent and recognize that his laboratory skills were too valuable to the Service to be wasted on this tiny island, allowing him to return to Washington and resume the work that he felt more urgently every time he glanced at the yellowing photograph of Bettie hanging in their makeshift home.

CHAPTER 2

THE *NIPPON MARU*

The ship appeared out of the fog at dawn, like a ghost made real. As it neared Angel Island, sailors hoisted a yellow flag, an international symbol that the ship carried diseased passengers on board. Only when it came closer could Marine Hospital Service personnel make out its name: the *Nippon Maru*. The ship, which originated in Hong Kong, was already notorious on both sides of the Pacific. It had languished in quarantine at both Yokohama and Honolulu after several of its passengers died of suspected plague on the open seas, but was ultimately cleared to sail on toward the United States. Now weeks behind schedule, it dropped anchor off the main cove of the island, once again tainted by an unexplained death on board.

A doctor from the Marine Hospital Service met the ship and learned that a Japanese woman had died, apparently of plague, two days before the steamer reached San Francisco and had been buried at sea. He then examined the lifeless body of another passenger, a Chinese man who had died the previous day from what appeared to be the same illness. He took tissue samples from the corpse and ordered it cremated, while the remaining fifty-five passengers were placed under quarantine on Angel Island. A team of Marine Hospital Service men boarded the ship and began washing down its surfaces with boiling hot water, intent on killing any traces of the unidentified disease, while another removed all the luggage and cargo and fumigated it with a mixture of steam and carbolic acid, destroying all clothing in the process.

Kinyoun, who had been the first American to study the newly discovered plague bacillus two years before, raced the tissue samples taken from the dead man to his laboratory, thrilled to once again put his research skills to work after weeks of self-doubt. There, he examined the cells under his microscope and began the slow work of growing them in a culture. Only then would he be able to determine how great a risk the men and women now in quarantine posed to the city. If plague had been on board and was spreading, then any one of the fifty-five passengers now in his custody would be capable of sparking an epidemic that could kill millions.

The following morning, an Italian crab fisherman by the name of Joseph Casarino discovered the bodies of two men floating face down in the water about an eighth of a mile east of Fort Point, a Civil War-era fortification at the mouth of the bay which in time would fall under the shadow of the Golden Gate Bridge. Casarino threw a rope over the bodies and towed them toward a small beach behind the nearby Fulton Iron Works. As he neared land, he noticed that the dead men wore uninflated life preservers bearing the name *Nippon Maru*, which by then was well-known throughout the city as a suspected plague ship. Fearing for his life, he left the bodies floating just offshore and alerted the city coroner, who paid him twenty dollars for his service.

At the city morgue, the coroner on duty began the grim work of inspecting the bloated corpses to determine the cause of death. Both men were wearing only their underwear when their bodies were found, with the shorter of the pair having apparently tied a bundle of his clothing around his neck, strongly suggesting they had intentionally jumped into the cold, shark-infested waters of the bay and were attempting to swim to shore when they died. An autopsy revealed that their lungs and stomachs were full of saltwater, indicating that the immediate cause of death was drowning. Yet the coroner suspected more. "In my mind there is no doubt that the men were infected with the plague," he told one of the city's papers. "I would not be surprised to learn that the men were driven from the steamer by some of their fellow passengers in steerage who were afraid of being tied up at the quarantine station." Dr. William Barbat, a member of the San Francisco Board of Health, took a sample of tissue from each of the bodies and without first conferring with Kinyoun announced the next day that after studying the specimens in his laboratory he was sure of the presence of bubonic plague, which had never before appeared in the United States.

Kinyoun objected, and loudly. Given the Marine Hospital Service's role in regulating all incoming sea and land traffic that originated outside of California, he alone had the authority to determine the risk that the passengers now sleeping on iron cots in the quarantine ward posed to the city. But more than that, he considered Barbat a scientist of far lower rank and skill whose opinion he was free to ignore. Not only had no definitive laboratory diagnosis of plague ever been made in such a short period of time, but the bodies of the drowned men were in such a deteriorated state after bobbing in the bay for at least twelve hours that all surviving tissue was unusable. Kinyoun's own tests conducted on tissue samples taken from the undisturbed body of the Chinese man who died aboard the *Nippon Maru* soon came back negative for the disease, leaving him to wonder how two diseased patients would have the strength to try to swim for freedom while a passenger free of plague had resigned to stay and die aboard the ship.

In his first important decision in San Francisco, Kinyoun fell back on his worst instincts. Unmoved by the opinions of local doctors that clashed with his own research, he announced that the detained passengers would be allowed to enter San Francisco once the fifteen-day quarantine period was over as long as they showed no symptoms of disease. When the Board of Health publicly questioned his findings, he was quick to resort to sarcasm, unconcerned that there might come a day when he may need its help. "I think there must be two kinds of bubonic plague, the real thing and the state quarantine plague," he quipped to a newspaper reporter. After Barbat took a ferry to Angel Island to complain in person, Kinyoun mocked his technical abilities and threatened to throw him into quarantine for handling specimens that he was unqualified to touch.

After fifteen days had passed without any signs of plague, the detained passengers formed lines and were led onto ferries to take them to San Francisco. Kinyoun stood watch on the dock, receiving handshakes and words of thanks from men and women as they passed on toward freedom. The fifty-five passengers who first walked into quarantine were joined by one addition, an infant named Margaret Francis Hill whose mother went into labor the day after she arrived on Angel Island and gave birth under Kinyoun's care in a makeshift delivery room. None of the passengers later came down with the disease, proving that Kinyoun's diagnosis was correct. Yet once again, he had put being right above anything else, destroying the possibility of making new allies only three weeks after he had arrived in a city he did not understand.

Six months later, an urgent bulletin arrived from Hawaii. Marine Hospital Service doctors stationed on the islands were the first to tell the outside world that bubonic plague had emerged and was spreading in Honolulu. Kinyoun knew then that his mission had changed. With San Francisco the most heavily trafficked port on the Pacific Coast and the main link between the United States and Hawaii, it was inevitable that the disease would be lurking in one of the hundreds of ships that were bound this way.

There was no room for error. If he failed to spot a single infected passenger, Kinyoun would hold himself responsible for the spread of death on an unimaginable scale. Not only was the city he glimpsed across the bay in danger, but a person carrying the disease could easily hop on one of the countless trains connecting San Francisco with the rest of a nation stretching across the continent. A train heading east would stop in every major city along its route, making it possible for one infected patient to scatter plague from Salt Lake City to Denver to Chicago and New York within the span of days, a speed never before seen in history and which would overwhelm any attempt at containment.

Yet with this news came the chance to reclaim what Kinyoun saw as his rightful position in Washington. Quickly spotting and preventing the disease from establishing itself in the country would cement in the public's mind the notion that laboratory science could save lives, accelerating the legitimacy of his profession and increasing his own prestige. A posting that Wyman had intended as punishment had become the primary line of defense against a disease that had never before reached North America. If he succeeded, Kinyoun would finally have redemption.

As the new century began, Kinyoun spent his days staring at the ships coming in through the Golden Gate from his perch on Angel Island, waiting. One of them would eventually bring a patient infected with plague, and he vowed to himself that he would be ready. He pored over every dispatch from Honolulu, where much of its Chinatown remained under quarantine, effectively turning one of its most populated districts into a jail. Kinyoun hoped the flurry of telegrams would offer some clues that would help him protect San Francisco. Instead, it soon became clear that the largest city in Hawaii was falling into chaos.

On January 20, firefighters in Honolulu set a small shack next to Kaumakapili Church ablaze, taking care to position their horse-drawn fire engine between the fire and the mammoth building whose twin Gothic spires towered over the city. An hour later, the winds unexpectedly shifted, sending burning embers flying over the most famous house of worship on the islands. Firemen watched in disbelief as smoke began pouring out of the top of the church, too high for their hoses to reach. Within minutes, the entire building was in flames, and became the center of a firestorm that quickly engulfed the neighborhood. The horses harnessed to the fire engine bolted in fear, leaving firemen with no way to douse the swirling flames.

Men scrambled through the inferno, dodging burning debris as the fire tore through the densely packed neighborhood. Panicked residents began dynamiting buildings over the objections of their owners, desperately hoping to create a firebreak. Amid the chaos, dozens of white Hawaiians rushed to the edge of Chinatown with axes and revolvers in hand, threatening to kill any Asian resident who tried to flee from the burning quarantine zone. Firecrackers exploding in abandoned buildings sparked rumors throughout the district that soldiers were gunning down men and women in their homes. Desperate families were trapped as the flames bore down on them, left with the choice between burning to death or getting shot or bludgeoned by men who feared plague.

Finally, at mid-afternoon, the military relented and allowed residents of Chinatown to escape the firestorm through a single exit. More than a thousand armed white Hawaiians lined King Street to stand guard as shocked refugees made their way downtown to the grounds of Kawaiaha'o Church, the former national church of the Hawaiian kingdom. There, they were issued tents and blankets and waited in silence as their former homes were reduced to ash. Health officials soon moved the residents of Chinatown to a former barrack in the hills far away from the city center. Over the following weeks, refugees from the district were required to take daily showers in front of doctors who were convinced that their filthy bodies would spread plague. The fire continued to burn on in Chinatown for another seventeen days before it was fully extinguished, leaving nothing but rubble behind.

In the coming weeks, no new cases of plague were discovered in Honolulu, leaving health officials content that the policy of fire had worked. For Kinyoun, however, his options seemed to narrow: either prevent the disease from establishing itself in San Francisco, or risk burning down the city in order to prevent the disease from infecting the nation.

CHAPTER 3

THE IMPERIAL CITY

If San Francisco seemed like a stranger to Joseph Kinyoun, that was to be expected. The city often seemed like a stranger to itself, unsure of its place in the new century.

Fifty years earlier it had been the epicenter of one of the greatest hysterias the world had ever seen. On January 24, 1848, a carpenter by the name of James Marshall spotted glittering flakes in the clear flowing waters of the American River near Coloma while building a sawmill for John Sutter, a Swiss immigrant who ruled over a fifty-thousand-acre fiefdom he called New Helvetia near what is now the city of Sacramento. Marshall gathered some of the material that caught his eye and rode on horseback through heavy rain to Sutter's Fort some fifty miles away. Once there, he took Sutter to a private room and told him to lock the door. He then revealed a rag he had hidden in his jacket; nestled inside were more than two ounces of shimmering dust. The men at the mill thought him crazy, he said, but he believed that it was gold. Marshall paced as Sutter consulted the entry on gold in a nearby *Encyclopedia Americana* and began experimenting on the material. He soon determined that it was indeed gold, with a purity of at least twenty-three carats—a nearly flawless composition rarely found in the natural world.

The men agreed to mention their finding to no one and left the next day for the sawmill, arriving just before sunset. Taking care not to draw attention to themselves, they walked along the sandy bank of the river, trying to determine whether Marshall could repeat his discovery. By nightfall they had collected an additional ounce without effort. The next morning, they again ventured out alone and found gold not only in the riverbed but in dried-up creeks and ravines twisting off it, in amounts so plentiful that Sutter was able to dislodge a solid lump weighing an ounce and a half with nothing more than a small knife he had in his pocket.

Despite their precautions, they soon discovered that they had been followed. A Native American who worked for Sutter had trailed them all morning, and that afternoon rushed into a clearing full of ranch hands while holding a nugget he'd pulled from the river above his head and shouting *"Oro! Oro!,"* the Spanish word for gold. His secret lost, Sutter begged the men to keep the discovery to themselves for six more weeks, giving him enough time to complete a flour mill then under construction in nearby Brighton that had already cost him $25,000, a sum equivalent to nearly $720,000 in today's dollars. Concealing the fact that gold nuggets were just lying there for the taking was beyond any man's capacity for self-censorship, however, and word soon leaked out beyond Sutter's realm, creating a golden myth of California that it would never shed.

San Francisco, then a city of less than a thousand people that had changed its name from Yerba Buena the year before, found itself forever changed. For more than two hundred years, the fog engulfing the Golden Gate had acted like a false door, masking the entrance to the bay from European explorers even as settlements as close as Monterey grew into cities. Now, with the discovery of gold, the world came rushing in. With its deep bay, the city became the hub of gold country, through which all the spoils and sins of sudden wealth flowed. The value of horses, tin pans, axes—anything that could be of use in extracting metal from the earth—shot up in value beyond all rationality. Saloons, hotels, banks and brothels sprouted along the hills around the bay, leaving a travel writer by the name of Bayard Taylor to say of San Francisco that it "seemed to accomplish in a day the growth of half a century."

It seemed that every able-bodied man disappeared from the city and raced into the gold fields for days at a time, consumed by the proximity of wealth and what it could bring. Identities built up over a lifetime shattered upon the news of Marshall's discovery, undone by the prospect of striking it rich. Family, friendships, responsibilities—gold drained the luster from everything that had previously seemed to matter and replaced it with the fever dreams of possibility. Even children were known to venture into the gold fields without supplies and come back after just one day with the modern equivalent of more than $250 worth of gold flakes in their hands.

By the fall of 1848, rumors of gold had traveled across the continent and reached New York. Skeptical of what seemed to be nothing more than tall tales, the *New York Herald* sent reporters to investigate. They came back with a story that declared that, compared to the wealth flowing through Californian streams, "the famous El Dorado was but a sand bank, the Arabian nights were tales of simplicity!" In December, President James Polk formally announced the discovery of gold to the nation, declaring in a speech to Congress that "the accounts of abundance of gold are of such an extraordinary character as would scarcely command belief were they not corroborated by the authentic reports of officers in the public service."

Across the country, farmers left their crops, captains abandoned their boats, and merchants closed their doors, all to head toward San Francisco and the gold fields that lay within reach of its bay. By the end of 1849, an estimated 100,000 Americans had set off for California, sparking what would become the largest mass migration in the country's history. The young men who left their homes to head west called themselves Argonauts, a nod to what they saw as their grand quest for glory in an uncharted land. In San Francisco, dozens of clipper ships heavy with prospective miners emerged each day from the fog, as if it were an invasion. One Illinois paper printed a gold miner's goodbye poem to his wife, in which he wrote,

Farewell, dear wife, keep up good cheer,
There's glittering scenes before me
You soon with me the wealth shall share
That lays in California.
I'll hunt the mountains, search the sand,
Through weather clear and stormy,
With shovel, spade, and sieve in hand,
Dig Gold in California.
The Sacramento's banks are lined,
"They" credibly inform me,
With metals of the richest kind—
I *must* see California.

Sutter, the man who ruled what is now Sacramento before Marshall's discovery, found himself overwhelmed by the number of Argonauts and their audacity. Gold seekers besieged his property, stealing even the heavy millstones used to grind grain. "By this sudden discovery of the gold, all my great plans were destroyed," he would later write. "Had I succeeded for a few years before the gold was discovered, I would have been the richest citizen on the Pacific shore; but it had to be different. Instead of being rich, I am ruined." Marshall, too, failed to reap the rewards of the boom he had created. Unable to complete the sawmill after all his workers abandoned him to search for gold, he proved unable to recreate his luck as a prospector, dying penniless in a small cabin near what is now known as Eldorado National Forest.

In the year following Marshall's discovery, San Francisco's population jumped above twenty-five thousand, and every new day crammed more people into a place that felt less like heaven and more like hell. Dogs, cats and pigs roamed thoroughfares choked with broken-down carts, filthy clothing, rotting vegetables and the carcasses of overworked horses. In the fall, rain turned the streets into a thick, muddy slop, leaving one French visitor to proclaim that "This is not a town, it is a quagmire." Despite the wealth flowing through it, San Francisco was a "nasty, dirty, slushy, raviney, sand-hilly place," according to one doctor who found gold and then left town as quickly as he could. If barroom fights or bandits didn't kill newly arrived Argonauts, then cholera could, with epidemics engulfing the city in 1850, 1852 and 1854 as waves of newly arrived gold seekers continued to dig water wells just one or two feet deep and without regard for the proximity of nearby latrines. All told, one in five gold seekers died within their first six months in San Francisco, according to estimates at the time.

The city's transient population made any semblance of sanitation an afterthought. In 1852, residents were still using the site of one of the few rudimentary hospitals that could be found within a hundred miles as a dumping ground, lining its square with what one visitor called "an immense pile of rubbish and filth of the worst description." When they weren't throwing it into public spaces, San Franciscans were discarding their trash into gaping holes which opened in the middle of poorly made roads that were often little more than dirt paths up and down its network of hills. City inspectors dumped buckets of chaparral, sand and flour into the pits in a vain effort to congeal them into a solid surface, yet the holes inevitably opened again, often requiring residents to walk the length of a city block to find a level place to cross the street.

San Francisco felt perpetually on the edge of destruction, a feeling kindled by an onslaught of seven major fires in a span of eighteen months. Still, those who were able to survive in this unconstrained land forged new identities as self-made men, willing to brave unnamed obstacles and make their fortunes—even if it was mainly luck they were counting on. They simply assumed that they were going to get rich, and their optimism was contagious. "Though I had but a single dollar in my pocket and no business whatsoever and did not know where I was going to get my next meal, I found myself saying to everybody I met, 'It is a glorious country!'" wrote Stephen Johnson Field, who left his law practice in Massachusetts to search for gold in California and was eventually nominated to the U.S. Supreme Court by Abraham Lincoln.

The belief that wealth was always just around the corner sustained the city from boom town through adolescence, with the gold mined from the nearby Sierra Nevada foothills slowly domesticating a place that remained famous for its vice. As the city grew richer, more ships clogged its docks, leaving a stew of South Americans, Australians, Chinese, Russians, Hawaiians, Europeans and Americans from the East Coast to amble along the streets. Countless bars and brothels blossomed in what was known as the Barbary Coast, a nine-block neighborhood that soon became a tourist draw on its own. "You are no longer in San Francisco, you are in Sailor town," one early guidebook to the city wrote. "It would be a courageous citizen, indeed, who would venture within its charmed precincts after nightfall unattended by a policeman, and it is the safest place on the coast in which a criminal can hide."

With an arduous months-long voyage that passed through the Panamanian jungle, around the iceberg-laden tip of South America, or by wagon train over the Rocky Mountains the only ways for the rest of the country to reach the state, California spent its first two decades in the Union as a land apart, independent both physically and mentally. It wasn't until 1869—twenty years after the first frenzy of the Gold Rush—that Central Pacific president Leland Stanford drove a spike made out of 17.6-carat gold into the tracks at Promontory Summit in what is now the state of Utah, completing the first transcontinental railroad. The link brought New York and the cities of the East Coast within a week's journey, opening up the glories of the state to a nation that remained in disbelief.

"We are so used to the California of the stage-coach, widely separated from the rest of the world, that we can hardly realize what the California of the railroad will be," wrote Henry George, an economist whose later work *Progress and Poverty* would help spur the Progressive Movement, in an 1868 essay. He envisioned a San Francisco with its own Astors and Vanderbilts, its own great museums, its own literature and its own artists—an explosion of culture that could only flourish in an environment of abundance.

"There is in the whole world no city—not even Constantinople, New Orleans, or Panama—which possesses equal advantages," he wrote. "From San Diego to the Columbia river, a stretch of over 1000 miles of coast, the bay of San Francisco is the only possible site for a great city. For the whole of the vast and rich country behind, this is the only gate to the sea. Not a settler in all the Pacific States and Territories but must pay San Francisco tribute; not an ounce of gold dug, a pound of ore smelted, a field gleaned, or a tree felled in all their thousands of square miles, but must, in a greater or less degree, add to her wealth . . . Considering these things, is it too much to say that this city of ours must become the first city of the continent; and is it too much to say that the first city of the continent must ultimately be the first city of the world? And when we remember the irresistible tendency of modern times to concentration— remember that New York, Paris and London are still growing faster than ever—where shall we set bounds to the future population and wealth of San Francisco; where find a parallel for the city which a century hence will *surround* this bay?"

By the turn of the twentieth century, San Francisco was home to one out of every four people who lived west of the Rockies and was the richest and most important port on the Pacific, as deeply tied to trade from Asia as to the East Coast. It reigned as the unquestioned cultural and financial capital of California, a state so overflowing with superlatives that it seemed blessed by God: home to the tallest trees, the deepest ports, the most fertile farmland and the wealthiest people.

The *Brooklyn Eagle* declared San Francisco the "most cosmopolitan town in the country outside of New York." Its banks handled more than one billion dollars each year, a figure greater than every other city in the West combined. The San Francisco Mint, a granite Greek Revival fortress standing at the corner of Fifth and Mission, held a third of the nation's gold deposits, a sum so monumental that it took some time before guards realized that $300,000 worth of gold had been stolen one New Year's Day. A few blocks away stood the Call Building, which at 310 feet loomed as the tallest structure west of Chicago and from whose porthole windows diners in the top-floor restaurant could look down upon the entire bay. At the foot of Market Street rose the tower of the Ferry Building, modeled on a Spanish cathedral, which was on its way to becoming the second busiest transportation hub in the world. In Golden Gate Park, workers were putting another coat of gleaming white paint on the Conservatory of Flowers, a Victorian jewel box which was one of the first public conservatories in North America.

"It was a city of romance and a gateway to adventure," wrote Will Irwin in a memoir of the city at the turn of the century. "It opened out on the mysterious Pacific, the untamed ocean; and through the Golden Gate entered China, Japan, the South Sea Island, Lower California, the west coast of Central America, Australia. There was a sprinkling too, of Alaska and Siberia. From his windows on Russian Hill one always saw something strange and suggestive creeping through the mists of the bay. It would be a South Sea Island brig, bringing in cope, to take out cottons and idols; a Chinese hunk after shark's livers; an old whaler, which seemed to drip oil, home from a year of cruising in the Arctic."

But for all its charms, San Francisco remained hollow, a town more rooted in façade than fact. Graft, corruption and self-interest were a part of the city's foundation, the natural consequence of a metropolis whose population believed in fate rather than skill. Nothing embodied this more than City Hall, which when it officially opened in 1897 was the largest municipal building west of Chicago. Its elaborate design, the product of twenty-five years of construction, was beautiful to behold, with a three-hundred-foot-high dome rising above the city's Hall of Records. Yet it was rotting from within.

"On taking possession of City Hall we found it in a most dilapidated condition and so filthy as to be almost beyond description," wrote John Barnett, the superintendent of public buildings, in a 1900 report. "The corridors were covered with the dirt of the ages; every closet in the building where dirt, ashes and rubbish could be stored was filled to overflowing; the rotunda and vestibule were coated with the original dirt, lime and mortar made in construction; the sub-basement was so filthy as to endanger the health of any person who was compelled to pass through it; several parts of it, which were below level, were filled with stagnant water; the leader pipes running to the sewer were broken in many places, and many of the sewer pipes opened directly into the sub-basement; the water closets and toilet rooms throughout the building were so unsanitary that the occupants of the building who had any regard for their health would not use them . . . the plastering in all of the corridors and in many of the rooms looked very much as if some person or persons had deliberately tried to remove it from the walls with a hatchet."

Stuck at a crossroads between its rough past and a new future in which gold was no longer plentiful, the city that confronted Kinyoun from across the bay was facing an uncomfortable reality in which white men could not easily find work, breeding a generation that felt cheated out of the riches once showered upon their grandfathers. All the while, men and women expecting the easy life continued to arrive from the East Coast, multiplying the number of the poor and frustrated.

"Even now, far and wide, people think of California as a region where wealth is not dependent on thirst, where one can somehow 'strike it rich' without that tedious attention to details and expenses which wears out life in effete regions such as Europe and the Eastern states," wrote David Starr Jordan, the founding president of Stanford University, in a widely read essay titled "California and the Californians." "San Francisco, by force of circumstances, has become the hopper into which fall incompetents from all the world, and from which few escape . . . The city contains more than four hundred thousand people. Of these, a vast number, thirty thousand to fifty thousand, it may be, have no real business in San Francisco. They live from hand to mouth, by odd jobs that might be better done by better people; and whatever their success in making a living, they swell the army of discontent, and confound all attempts to solve industrial problems."

Still, the every-man-for-himself spirit of the gold rush lingered on, halting any proposed solutions before they could be launched. The city could not even bring itself to fund its public health department, believing that it was a waste of money at best and a swindle at worst. As its population doubled between 1870 and 1885, San Francisco's spending on sanitation, hospitals and other forms of medical care and prevention fell by 20 percent, leaving it a big city with the festering health issues of a frontier boomtown. "There is not, and never has been, a noble generosity in California," one physician wrote at the time. Those who did fall ill and had little means could expect to "languish in boarding houses and private homes, often badly cared for . . . until death mercifully comes to their relief."

In response to the palpable sense of anger among its white citizens, Mayor James D. Phelan cast the city's Asian immigrants as its chief problem. Racism and bigotry had been a part of California since the first Spanish encounters with natives in the sixteenth century; the rising influence of the new science of anthropology and the 1859 publication of Darwin's *On the Origin of Species* gave prejudice a scientific veneer and greater urgency. Taking their cue from Darwin's notion of the survival of the fittest, scientists began envisioning race as nothing less than a battle for the future. In his influential work *On the Unity of Mankind,* German physician Johann Blumenbach identified five major species of humanity, each of which possessed what he called unalterable physical and moral traits. Caucasians, he posited, were the closest to God, with strong, beautiful bodies "not stained with pigment." He lumped together all Asians into a lesser species he termed Mongolian, who were marked by small skulls—a sign of diminished intellect and depraved morals—and yellow skin, which suggested laziness.

In America, the idea that Asians were both wily and brutish took hold. The historian Hubert Bancroft noted in his book *Mongolianism in America* that "It was quite amusing to see [Chinese men] here and there and everywhere, and to show them to strangers as one of the many unique features California could boast. It put one in quite good humor with one's self to watch them waddling under the springy pole sustaining at either end a huge and heavily laden basket; it made one quite feel one's superiority to see these queer little specimens of petrified progress, to listen to their high-keyed strains of feline conversation, and notice all their cunning curiosity and barbaric artlessness."

The backbreaking demands of building the transcontinental railroad led railroad companies first to hire Chinese workers in California, and then to import as many as fifteen thousand men directly from China. By 1867, approximately 90 percent of all laborers laying track and tunneling through the mountains were Chinese, doing work that white men refused to do. "A large majority of the white laboring class on the Pacific Coast find most profitable and congenial employment in mining and agricultural pursuits, than in railroad work," Leland Stanford told Congress. "The greater portion of the laborers employed by us are Chinese . . . without them it would be impossible to complete the western portion of this great national enterprise."

The willingness of the Chinese who remained after the railroad was completed to work for low wages led the Workingmen's Party, headed by a former sailor and gifted orator by the name of Denis Kearney, to form vengeful mobs in the 1870s that burned and plundered Chinese settlements from Seattle to San Diego. In Los Angeles, then a lawless outpost of approximately six thousand people, the city's two newspapers ran near-daily editorials condemning the roughly 175 Chinese residents of the city as dirty and inferior. After a popular saloon owner named Robert Thompson was killed in a shootout between two police officers and members of a Chinese gang in 1871, a mob of nearly 500 white men surrounded a building housing the suspected shooters and dragged them outside. There, at a makeshift gallows constructed at John Goller's wagon shop, seventeen men were lynched, their bodies hanging from the shop's portico and from the edges of nearby freight wagons. By morning, 10 percent of the city's Chinese population was dead. Only one of the victims was later thought to have been involved in the gunfight which sparked the massacre.

Kearney went on a national speaking tour soon after, punctuating his speeches with calls for "bullets to replace ballots" if white business owners continued to employ the Chinese, and once threatened to block the Golden Gate with the dead bodies of Chinese immigrants. "I made up my mind that if our civilization—California civilization—was to continue, Chinese immigration must be stopped," he thundered, before ending his speech with the rallying cry, "The Chinese must go."

Mayor Phelan, himself the son of an Irish immigrant and later a candidate for the U.S. Senate on a platform pledging to "Keep California White," tried to put Kearney's sentiments into municipal action. Though he presided over a city that cared little for government and even less for taxes, he argued that the only way forward for the white working class was for the city to issue bonds to fund the construction of public works projects which would put it on a par with those towns on the East Coast that many had fled, while excluding Asians from civic and economic life.

"The rough work of the building of a city has been successfully accomplished in San Francisco. The forest, as it were, has been cleared, the land has been tilled, the promise is abundant. We must bank on that," Phelan wrote in a Christmas Day message in 1897. "We are far enough away from the great cities of the East to develop an individuality, and that very remoteness makes it incumbent upon us to work out our own salvation."

Wong Chut King knew that to live in San Francisco was to remain in the shadows. At the age of forty-one, he had spent the majority of the last two decades of his life in dank, dark rooms, spending as little as he could to ensure his survival. Whatever money he did manage to keep from his job at a rat-infested lumberyard on Pacific Street he sent back to his wife and parents in his native village of Bei Keng, a tiny hamlet located in the southwest corner of China's Guangdong province.

He had arrived in California—known in his native Cantonese as Gum Shan, or the Gold Mountain—in the mid-1880s, most likely having been recruited from his village by a labor broker who covered the cost of the long trip across the Pacific to Canada. Once there, he made his way across the unguarded border and headed south toward San Francisco. He traveled by foot and wagon along the coast, unnerved by the towering redwoods—taller than any structure he had ever seen—rising above him, and felt the chill of the Pacific seep into his bones as he lay alone at night, trying to remember the warm, humid air flowing off the rivers at home. He expected a hard life once he reached the city, and he soon found it.

The first known Chinese immigrants had reached California during the frenzy of the Gold Rush in 1849, and within five years there were forty thousand Chinese living in the state. The influx of newcomers, with foreign habits and their foreign tongues, prompted lawmakers in some of the first sessions of the new state legislature to pass a series of discriminatory acts targeting Asians. The Chinese Exclusion Act—the first major law to restrict immigration into the United States—passed in 1882, prompted by fears among white Americans that an influx of Chinese laborers was pushing wages down. Ten years later, California congressman Thomas Geary introduced the Geary Act, which when passed extended the Chinese Exclusion Act

by ten years and required all Chinese residents to carry a certificate
of residence at all times or face deportation or a year of hard labor.

With even those who had once entered the country legally banned
from becoming citizens or owning property, Chinese residents of
San Francisco crammed into twelve blocks surrounding Portsmouth
Square, a plaza which stood at the center of the original Spanish
settlement of Yerba Buena. There, within yards of the site where
the first American flag in the city was raised, Chinese immigrants
created a self-contained neighborhood that seemed transported from
the other side of the world. Chinese characters painted in black
and gold hung from buildings, sharing space with lanterns dangling
from slanting wooden balconies. Gates decorated with dragons or
lions designed to ward off ghosts and other evil spirits enclosed
makeshift courtyards. Second-floor brothels and opium dens run by
tongs—secret societies that often overlapped with the underworld—
catered to the weaknesses of a population that was almost entirely
male, and became a draw for white tourists and sailors. Largely
ignored by white politicians, the neighborhood fell under the power
of what became known as the Chinese Six Companies, an umbrella
organization run by wealthier and better-educated immigrants who
banded together for mutual aid and protection.

For many, their adventure to California was meant to be short-
lived, a chance to strike it rich and then return to their villages
wealthy men. Wong, like many of these men, walked the streets of
San Francisco with the top of his head shaved and a long, braided
ponytail known as a queue trailing down his back, a symbol of loyalty to the emperor and a necessity for any man wishing to return
to China. With only enough money to survive, he faced most days
clad in a long, flowing black shirt and black pants, the darkness of
the cloth hiding its grime. Like most men in Chinatown, he could
neither read nor write, leaving him reliant on his imagination to
keep up with the daily life of his family as it unspooled back at
home. On days when his loneliness seemed more than he could
bear, Wong spent hours in cramped theaters watching long-winded

reenactments of traditional Chinese dramas, aching for anything that offered a sense of familiarity while he was exiled on the other side of the world.

He lived in the Globe Hotel, located at the corner of Dupont and Jackson, a ramshackle building known throughout the city for the illegal gambling which took place within its narrow rooms. Nearly three hundred people packed into the four-story structure, creating a notorious tenement that, upon a tour of the establishment, left the *San Francisco Chronicle* to report, "like rats in a barrel, poor, unwashed heathens crowd together in little cubby-holes." With nowhere else to go, residents throughout Chinatown built wooden additions onto the sides of buildings, on rooftops, and in hand-dug basements that in some cases burrowed into the foundation of the structure next door. White property owners cared little about the modifications to their tumble-down buildings, happy to collect the exorbitant monthly rents they were able to charge and buoyed by leases that put all responsibility for upkeep on the residents' shoulders. "Property leased to Chinamen in San Francisco is among the most productive in the city, and 30,000 Chinese pay annually one million dollars in rents alone," noted the *San Francisco Chronicle*. The few white faces that could be seen in the neighborhood belonged to either tourists or policemen, all of whom were drawn to the district's reputation for lawlessness.

Even in a place known for its filth, Wong's quarters were repellent. His room was located beneath the sidewalk in a space dug out from the original cellar. Liquid from an underground cesspool leaked through the wooden boards lining the room, creating a smell so pungent as to make visitors gag upon entry. A small open pit functioned as his only toilet. He shared his bed with two or three roommates, each man sleeping on the hard wooden mattress in turn. A solid wooden block served as his pillow. Sticks of burning incense and an untouched glass of wine—meant to curry favor with the gods of health and medicine—sat on a dirty crate in the middle of the room. Above it ran the pipe of an unused sewer line, home to a nest of rats that scampered in the shadows cast by a flickering oil lamp. Dreams, when they did come, allowed him to gaze upon the face of his wife and family as they praised him for his sacrifices, a thought that broke the misery of his life.

Wong continued to work and send remittances to his village until late February of 1900, when he noticed a lump in his right groin that was painful to the touch. It soon became difficult to move his leg or urinate without agony. Fearful that he had contracted a venereal disease that would bring him shame, he consulted a prominent physician, Wong Woo, in his office at 766 Clay Street. The doctor confirmed his suspicions and recommended salty foods and cooling herbs to drain the lump, following the traditional Chinese medical approach that regarded illness as a sign of disharmony in the body. Wong returned to his subterranean room and prayed, hoping that his indiscretions would be forgiven by the god Zhao Shen, who ruled over family life and recommended punishment to the magistrates in charge of the underworld.

Over the next few days, his temperature climbed and he began to lose control of his body, spending his few waking moments alternating between vomiting, diarrhea and delusions. As it became clear that Wong was nearing death, the men sharing his living quarters took action. Cantonese tradition carried a marked aversion to death, lest one become tainted by so-called killing airs that led to bad luck. The practice dated back to the biblical-era Han dynasty and confounded native-born Americans. "Nearly every week the police discover some wretched unfortunate that has been left to die in an underground den by unnatural relatives or friends," wrote *Cosmopolitan* magazine. "Medical attention or proper care he will get none. Slow starvation in a noisome cellar, in the hour of thick darkness, with vermin swarming over the helpless sufferer—such is the fate that has befallen many a poor creature in Chinatown."

Wong's roommates carried his still-breathing body to a coffin shop two blocks away. There, he was placed in one of the "halls of tranquility" that Chinese funeral homes maintained for the gravely ill, pungent rooms in which the dying were often placed next to open coffins and the bodies of unburied dead as they waited for the inevitable. There he lay until he died on the afternoon of March 6, 1900, a passing altogether unremarkable in a city that had never noticed his existence.

The shop's owner, Wing Sun, wrapped the body in canvas and prepared a simple pine coffin for burial and eventual retrieval. Funeral home directors were responsible for maintaining the custom of shipping the bones of Chinese immigrants back to their native villages following total decomposition of the flesh. Once back in China, their remains would be reburied in a family plot, allowing the dead to take their place among their ancestors and be worshiped by the living. Those whose bodies were mutilated or whose bones did not return to their homeland were believed to roam the earth as ghosts, haunting those who had prevented their journey into the afterlife. As a result, family members or friends routinely refused to consent to autopsies or other medical procedures that violated the body, bound by the fear that in doing so they would bring upon themselves the wrath of their departed loved ones.

An assistant city health officer by the name of Frank Wilson arrived at the coffin shop later that evening as part of his normal rounds, in which he issued burial permits for a fee of three dollars each. Wilson had recently drawn the ire of the acting police chief for issuing death certificates that even he admitted were mostly guesswork, and with the help of an interpreter examined Wong's body with a thoroughness that was unusual for a man who routinely chalked up benign deaths to nonexistent bullet and knife wounds. He soon discovered an egg-shaped black lump on the right groin that he would have never found if he had not been afraid of losing his job. Alarmed by what he saw, Wilson called in his supervisor, Aloysius O'Brien. O'Brien was a surgeon and graduate of the University of California who had been recently reinstated to his position and, like Wilson, was eager to prove his worth. He inspected the body and instinctively stepped back in fear. There, on the dead man's groin, was what appeared to be an infected lymph node swollen with blood—a textbook example of a bubo, which gives bubonic plague its name.

Despite the late hour, the men summoned William Kellogg, who had become the city's first bacteriologist just two months before. Kellogg rushed to the coffin shop and took samples from the dead man's lymph nodes, taking care to disinfect every instrument that touched the body. Everything before him suggested that the disease had slipped into the city, yet he was hesitant to act. Mindful of the *Nippon Maru* incident six months before, he resisted making an official diagnosis that, if proven wrong, would turn the city against him and surely lead to his firing. He instead readied tissue samples to take across the bay to Angel Island, where Kinyoun would have the responsibility of announcing to the world that plague had reached American shores.

At an emergency Board of Health meeting late that night, spooked health officials took the unprecedented step of imposing what they called a "precautionary" quarantine of Chinatown, essentially sealing a neighborhood that contained nearly 20 percent of the city's residents. The best they could hope for was that Wong's death was just a fluke—one diseased man who had somehow bypassed Kinyoun's watchful officers, not a harbinger of worse things to come.

As Kellogg raced toward the dock, the still of the night was broken by dozens of policemen assembling around the borders of Chinatown. There, lit by moonlight and gas lamps, they unspooled rope and strung it around the district, hoping that it would help curtail the spread of a disease that no one knew how to defeat. San Francisco had long known that plague was a possibility; now it faced an outbreak that could mean the city's end.

CHAPTER 4

CRIMINAL IDIOCY

B y sunrise twenty thousand men and women were trapped.
Residents of Chinatown awoke to find ropes and policemen
lining the perimeter of the twelve-block district, sealing nearly all of
the city's Asian population inside a boundary drawn by Broadway,
Kearny, California and Stockton streets. Angry crowds made up of
cooks, launderers and porters trying to reach their jobs crammed
against the police lines at dawn. Their protests echoed through the
neighborhood, stirring others from their beds. The most desperate
for work attempted to duck under the rope and make a break for
it, only to be stopped by batons. Small teams of police officers periodically rushed deep into Chinatown and returned escorting white
people who had found themselves on the wrong side of the blockade
when the sun came up.

Rumors raced through the district that health officials planned
to burn all of Chinatown to the ground with its residents trapped
inside, just as had been narrowly avoided in Honolulu. Men clam-
bered across rooftops and down into the sewer system, seeking any
path to freedom. Those who escaped the quarantine found that their
lot had hardly improved. Barred from boarding steamers leaving the
city, Chinese residents hid in private homes or jumped into small

boats and rowed into the fog of the bay, desperate to evade health officers.

Policemen accompanied Board of Health inspectors into Chinatown, where they attempted to reconstruct the last days of Wong's life. Little information was known about the man, leaving doctors with the feeling that they were chasing a ghost. As he had no known associates or friends, health officials canvassed the neighborhood, treating every person and building as suspect. At the Globe Hotel, workers sprayed formaldehyde in all of its rooms until the smell seeped into the floors, while the coffin shop where Wong's body had been discovered was fumigated and closed.

White physicians went door to door, searching for anyone who showed signs of infection. The noxious chemical smell wafting through the neighborhood further disoriented residents of Chinatown, many of whom had fled outbreaks in their villages and had more experience with plague than the white authorities who now encircled them. In their homeland, the disease was often seen as a divine punishment that required raucous processions to frighten away evil spirits with the sounds of drums and fireworks. Instead, they found themselves isolated, unable to escape either the disease or the white men they did not trust or understand.

With the Chinese imprisoned, the rhythms of San Francisco fell into chaos. Every cable car line running through Chinatown was suspended, creating a twelve-block obstacle to anyone traveling near downtown. Officials at the Customs House on Battery Street refused to issue clean bills of health to ships leaving the city for other ports, bringing the normal pandemonium of the piers to a standstill. Even routine shipping paperwork at the office stalled, with all the federal government's Chinese translators stuck in Chinatown. The same story played out across the paralyzed city, as if San Francisco was an animal trapped in tar. The chef at the Palace Hotel waited in vain for more than a dozen Chinese cooks, leaving the restaurant unable to serve its guests. In well-to-do private homes, breakfast tables went empty and soiled laundry piled up. Angry white employers overwhelmed the telephone switchboard in Chinatown, trying to track down the men and women they had come to rely on.

Few white San Franciscans feared that they were in any danger themselves, trusting instead in misguided notions that plague could only flourish in hot climates, and even then only among those who ate rice instead of a more muscular European diet centered on meat. This racist belief reached the highest stations, with W. K. Reypen, the Surgeon General of the Navy, telling a reporter that "The climatic conditions of the United States preclude the possibility of the plague ever getting within this country. It is a disease peculiar to the Orient, and seldom, if ever attacks Europeans . . . There is absolutely no danger of the plague ever getting here." Even those who could admit that plague might appear in Chinatown were adamant that it did not pose a threat to the city at large. "When these diseases appear they prove to be largely racial, as this plague is, and experience with it proves that Occidental races are but little subject to it. They have their own racial diseases to admonish them that they are mortal and must not crowd together too closely," noted the *San Francisco Call* in an editorial.

The city's newspapers immediately called the scare nothing but a ploy by the Board of Health to receive more funding, with the *San Francisco Chronicle* leading the charge. "In its desire to tighten the city into giving it the desired appropriation, with increased patronage, the board had caused the entire Chinese quarter to be blockaded," the paper announced, under the headline, "Nothing But a Suspicion: Criminal Idiocy of the Phelan Health Board." The *Call*, meanwhile, warned that the quarantine could derail the city's economy and accused Mayor Phelan of conjuring up the disease as a feint to grab more power. "There is no bubonic plague in San Francisco," the paper argued. "The most dangerous plague which threatens San Francisco is not of the bubonic type. A plague of politics brought to the city by a Mayor whose chief characteristic is to bargain and

barter in the powers given him by the new charter and by him transmitted to a Board of Health which has scandalized the community
by its extravagance and inefficiency, is the malady which not only
menaces the commercial interests, the prosperity and future of the
city, but is striking at the very foundation of its government."

In another time, in another city, charging an elected mayor with
inventing an outbreak of bubonic plague in order to secure more tax
dollars would seem preposterous. But in San Francisco, a town largely
created and populated by men and women driven to abandon their
previous lives in hopes of becoming rich, nothing seemed too low to
contemplate. Corruption drifted through the city as easily as the afternoon fog, touching every office in its wake. To live in San Francisco
required training oneself to keep an eye out for the next potential
swindle, to learn how to spot a fake before anyone else. Once city
officials began allowing cable cars—empty but for a few policemen
charged with keeping anyone in the quarantine zone from boarding—
to run through Chinatown the day after the blockade went up, the
most cynical in the city saw an admission that the fear of spreading the
germs of the so-called infected district was just for show.

And after all, the papers argued, if this was truly an outbreak, why
hadn't health authorities found more victims? "All I wish to say is
that if this Chinese had died of the plague every physician in the
city would have all he could do in the infected quarter. The germs
of the plague multiply by millions of millions in a very few hours,"
said Dr. E. O. Jellinek, whom the *Chronicle* called an expert in bacteriology and the plague, though his exact qualifications were left
unspecified. "However, days have passed and there are no more cases
reported. Besides, the body of this man bore none of the plague's
characteristic features and I would feel safe in saying that the fear
would be foolish as this quarantine is now unnecessary."

The one man who could determine whether a quarantine was
needed sat five miles away in a windblown island laboratory that

was still far beneath his standards, unaware until it was too late that anything had gone wrong. Kellogg arrived at Angel Island at dusk carrying samples of tissue taken from the body from Wong Chut King as the first ropes were being strung up around Chinatown. He greeted Kinyoun and filled him in on the possible buboes found on the dead man in nearly the same breath.

Kinyoun took the samples and hustled to his laboratory, where he began the grim process of determining whether the scenario that haunted his nightmares had become real. First, he peered at the cells through the microscope, looking for the distinctive rod-shaped bacillus. Once he confirmed its presence, he separated a part of the tissue sample and divided it into syringes which he injected into two guinea pigs, a rat and a monkey which he kept in cages in his laboratory. Should the animals develop the same symptoms as the dead man over the next few days, it would be powerful evidence that the plague was real and could spread. Once this was done, he examined the remaining material collected from Wong Chut King's body, hoping to isolate a selection of bacteria cells that he could grow in a culture in order to confirm the identity of the disease.

He was among the few doctors in the world who knew enough about the disease to even attempt to regrow it in a laboratory. The bacillus responsible for plague, now known as *Yersinia pestis*, had been identified just six years before. This discovery was one of the most notable achievements in the still-young field of bacteriology, and yet it cratered the reputation of one of the field's early stars.

In May of 1894, the Japanese government sent a team headed by Shibasaburo Kitasato—who, alongside Robert Koch in Berlin, had conducted the diphtheria research that had amazed Kinyoun, and whose brilliance would eventually lead the Emperor of Japan to grant him the title of baron—to Hong Kong to research the outbreak of plague decimating the city. Nearly half of the 100,000 residents had fled, leaving the roadways deserted and the harbor nearly empty. Great piles of dead rats lay untouched in infected areas, casting a stench of death that hung like a warning over the city and could be picked up from miles away. Within two days of his arrival, Kitasato was at work in a modern laboratory provided by the government, built in a former police station which had been converted into a plague hospital. There, with six assistants on hand, he searched for the organism behind the wave of disease spilling through the city, which threatened to leave Hong Kong nothing but a ruin.

A few weeks after Kitasato arrived, a Swiss-born French researcher by the name of Alexandre Yersin entered the city without fanfare. Like Kitasato, Yersin had studied at Koch's laboratory in Berlin, but after publishing a few landmark papers he left behind a promising career to travel alone to the newly united French colony of Indochina, hoping to follow in the footsteps of his hero, the British explorer David Livingstone. Short, shy and solitary by nature, Yersin preferred experimenting with the new technologies of radio and photography to the company of people, and adopted the peculiar habit of never using his first name if he could help it. He was only allowed into Hong Kong on the recommendation of one of his former mentors, Louis Pasteur, whom he had once dazzled with his accounts of wandering through present-day Vietnam. Once in the city, he spoke rarely, knowing only a handful of English words and possessing no desire to learn more.

Alone, without facilities, housing or government support, Yersin began his own experiments with a microscope and portable sterilizer, searching, like Kitasato, for the elusive cause of plague. He built a straw hut that functioned as both his laboratory and shelter and petitioned the government for cadavers for research. After being denied, he found more success by bribing sailors who were carting plague-infected bodies to cemeteries. Though Yersin knew Kitasato socially, he spoke to the man just a handful of times, conversing in their shared tongue of German. Both men were well aware that the other was pursuing the same goal, and a quiet rivalry developed between the two.

Yersin attended one autopsy conducted by Kitasato, and was struck by the fact that he was concentrating his attention on the

cadaver's blood, rather than on the buboes in the groin and armpits. Yersin, by contrast, focused almost exclusively on the swollen
buboes pocking the dead, a decision that soon proved fruitful. On
June 20, he wrote the first description of the bacterium responsible for killing millions since antiquity. "The pulp of the bubo, in
every case, was filled with a thick puree of short, thick bacilli with
rounded ends . . . One can recover a great amount from the buboes
and lymph nodes of the diseased. The blood also contains them but
not in such great numbers and only in very grave and deadly cases."
Mice, rats and guinea pigs injected with diseased tissues died two
to five days after infection, he reported. The location of the bubo
did not seem to matter, he found, as tissue extracted from various
organs all yielded the same quantity of bacilli, a stark sign of how
thoroughly plague consumed the human body.

Kitasato, for all of his material advantages, was unable to pinpoint
the plague bacillus as rapidly, sharing the results of his research only
in mid-August. Though his observations were similar enough to
Yersin's that the two men shared recognition for the discovery during their lifetimes, Kitasato made several telling errors in describing
the plague bacillus, which led to whispers among his contemporaries
that his cultures had been at least partly contaminated. Researchers following in Kitasato's footsteps the following year realized that,
on at least one occasion, the lion of Japanese research had instead
isolated the bacterium responsible for causing pneumonia, remark-
ably similar in shape and size to that behind the more devastating
disease. A proud man who hoped to return to his home country and
open a research institute bearing his name, Kitasato refused to admit
his error until 1899, when plague reached the Japanese port city of
Kobe, and then did so only privately. He conceded to a team of doctors hoping to forestall the epidemic that he had been mistaken, but
continued to insist that the culture in question was not pneumonia
but another, still-unidentified bacterium associated with plague.

Though driven by a need for medical certainty that made him
look to disprove the research of others as much as to conduct trials

of his own, Kinyoun accepted Kitasato's errors without judgment, still mesmerized by the older man's research into diphtheria, which had saved the lives of countless children. Kinyoun maintained a friendship with him for the remainder of his life, humbled to be in the presence of one of the few men he considered his intellectual superior. Kitasato, in turn, shared samples of *Yersinia pestis* with Kinyoun, making him the first American to study the bacterium. Long before he came to San Francisco, Kinyoun had spent hours in conversations with Kitasato, questioning him on every aspect of the plague epidemic in Hong Kong.

It was because of these talks that Kinyoun was perhaps the only person on the West Coast, and one of a handful in the entire country, who truly understood the progress of the disease he was fighting. A single infected patient arriving in a new city didn't spark a wide epidemic, he learned; the disease instead seeped slowly into the marrow of a city, only exploding out of a small zone once it had thoroughly established itself. The mechanism by which plague traveled from person to person was not yet fully known, however, leaving doctors grasping for ways to halt its spread or eliminate it completely.

Medicine at the time could only detail the methodical way in which plague consumed the body. After penetrating the skin of a human, the bacterium would begin to rapidly multiply, as if intent on overwhelming the body's defenses through sheer numbers. The bacteria were found to double within the human body within two hours, and then double again every two hours thereafter. White blood cells, the body's natural defenses, would soon be rendered helpless as the plague bacteria developed antigens that allowed them to overrun the lymphatic system. Within a week, patients infected with the disease would develop a bubo laden with as much as 100 billion plague bacteria per gram of tissue and fall into a stupor. The appearance of a bubo was an all but certain sign of death, with nearly all patients dying of organ failure within five days after one emerged on their body.

Modern scientists now understand that *Yersinia pestis* seems designed to kill. The bacterium has the ability to detect temperature around it, and once it is in an environment around the human body's resting state of 98.6 Fahrenheit it begins to modify the structure of a molecule in its outer membrane in an effort to mask itself from the immune system. The bacterium then moves toward the lymph nodes and destroys protective white blood cells known as macrophages by injecting toxins into them. Once inside the lymph nodes, *Y. pestis* releases a molecule called yersiniabactin which scours the bloodstream for iron, allowing the bacterium to replicate further while pushing its victim into an anemic stupor. The lymph nodes begin to swell, forming buboes, and the overabundance of bacteria in the bloodstream soon sends the body into septic shock, leading to abnormal blood clotting and organ failure.

While physicians knew the progression of the disease at the turn of the twentieth century, antibiotics, which might halt it as it ransacked a body, had yet to be developed. Instead, isolating a patient with the disease was the closest thing that medicine had to a cure. As Kinyoun readied the culture of cells, he knew that he was racing time. It was only by chance that the police had come across Wong Chut's body; perhaps other men and women had succumbed to plague over the last few months or years without notice, shortening the window that Kinyoun had before the disease was so well-established that all of San Francisco was at risk.

From nearly the moment he received the samples from Wong Chut's body, Kinyoun found himself thrust into a world for which he was uniquely unsuited. Used to the safe confines of his laboratory, he now faced a city that had no patience for a man who valued certitude over speed. His pride made him unable to consult with others who might offer guidance on how to smooth the political edges of his task; his lack of social graces left him with no network to draw on should he need it.

Even his fastidious routines—so useful in the pursuit of scientific truth—would soon be criticized, as the anxious city found itself unwilling to reconcile the methodical pace of the new era of science with the hourly demands of modern life. With few acquaintances and no close friends in the city, Kinyoun had no one to confide in. "I would like very much indeed to have some congenial spirit with whom to commune and hear out my worries, who would be a little closer than twenty-five hundred miles away," Kinyoun lamented in a letter to a friend in Washington.

Forty-eight hours after the quarantine was put in place, Phelan called an emergency midday meeting of the Board of Health. There, Kellogg announced that although Kinyoun's tests would not be conclusive for at least another day, "I inspected the inoculated animals today at Angel Island and found no indication of infection from the cultures injected, and I do not think now that the case is one of plague. Unless the animals die there will be nothing more to do; the incident will be closed."

With no input from Kinyoun, and with no one willing to wait until the test which could determine that the fate of the city was fully concluded, the Board of Health voted unanimously to lift the quarantine. Outside, Mayor Phelan proclaimed that the board had been justified in its decision to impose a temporary quarantine despite the disruptions that it caused, due to the city's position as the first line of defense against the "Asiatic infection to which San Francisco is constantly exposed." Phelan, who would later be forced to admit that he owned buildings in Chinatown from which he extracted exorbitant rents, then continued, "As to the objections and suits by the Chinese, I desire to say that they are fortunate, with the unclean bits of their coolies and their filthy hovels, to be permitted to remain within the corporate limits of any American city. In an economic sense their presence has been, and is, a great injury to the working classes, and in a sanitary sense they are a constant menace to the public health."

Within hours, the ropes encircling Chinatown were cut down,

sending hundreds of Chinese residents rushing out of the quarter to their jobs, where they hoped to confirm that they were still employed. Trash collectors making their first forays into the district for days found streets thick with spoiled meat and rotting vegetables. Hoping to prevent the city from imposing a similar quarantine in the future, Chinese merchants and the powerful Chinese Six Companies pressed for reimbursement for the hours their businesses had been forced to close and the merchandise that had expired. "If we do not protest and demand compensation, the Americans will only treat us even more cruelly," the Chinese-language newspaper *China West Daily* argued.

Lost amid the relief spreading through the city, Kinyoun was now the sole person left seeking the true cause of Wong Chut's death. His refusal to call off his tests made him a target for those in the city hoping to quash all mentions of plague. In a damaging blow to his pride, the *Chronicle* reported that "the quarantine officer is said to have one time diagnosed the germs of pneumonia as those of the black plague," misattributing Kitasato's error to Kinyoun. Not content with undercutting Kinyoun personally, the paper then mocked his methods, suggesting in an editorial that he needed to add a parrot into his menagerie for entertainment value alone. At least then one animal would "have been able to tell how it felt to have a lot of germs from a dead Chinese injected into his veins, and until the germs and starvation causes death, if the experiment resulted that way, the parrot might have joined forces with the monkey and made things interesting in the death cell," it joked.

Uncharacteristically quiet in the face of personal attacks, Kinyoun kept to himself at Angel Island, away from the din of a city that he was starting to loathe. He continually checked on the status of the animals in his care, looking for any sign that might calm his nerves despite the evidence of plague bacilli he had found in Wong Chut's tissue sample. His communication with the outside world consisted mainly of telegrams he sent to Washington, keeping Surgeon General Wyman up to date on the status of his research. Yet, owing to the continued friction between the men, all correspondence traveled through James Gassaway, the surgeon in charge of the Marine Hospital Service in San Francisco.

Wyman rarely responded to Kinyoun by name, maintaining an icy distance which gnawed at his already wounded pride. Rather than traveling out to San Francisco himself, the Surgeon General oversaw the Marine Hospital Service's response to plague from his perch in Washington. He ordered a lieutenant to board the first train from New Orleans to San Francisco, and, once the man arrived, sent him on a mission up the coast, stopping at every port and inquiring about possible infections.

Kinyoun saw the flurry of telegrams as a sign of a man unwilling or unable to face the backlash of a frightened city in person, and, on a night when he could not sleep, confided to Lizzie that he expected the situation to get worse soon. The day after the quarantine around Chinatown was lifted, Kinyoun awoke to discover his laboratory animals lying dead in their cages. He performed autopsies on each one, finding massive amounts of inflammation and bacilli that he identified as plague.

There was now no doubt in his mind that the disease he most feared was festering in the city, and he suspected that Wong Chut King was not its first victim—nor would he be its last.

CHAPTER 5

FAULT LINES

The confirmation that plague was now in San Francisco was largely ignored by those who desperately wanted it to be otherwise.

Physicians on the Board of Health refused to accept Kinyoun's findings, fearful that any acknowledgment of the disease would narrow their city's future. Reporters simply mocked him and amused themselves by implying that he had killed the animals himself out of impatience and greed. The deaths most likely came "as a result of neglect and the emaciation that follows close confinement and too persistent attention from eager bacteriologists," according to the *San Francisco Chronicle*. Other papers ran editorial cartoons depicting Kinyoun's inoculated animals picking the locks of the city treasury, a particularly stinging rebuke for a man who prided himself on his thrift.

Nor did Kinyoun find what should have been his natural allies in Washington. In an article published in January, shortly before the discovery of the disease in San Francisco, Wyman had expressed his skepticism that plague would ever pose a significant danger to the United States or Europe. "It seems impossible that the plague should ever again ravage the earth as in previous cities," Wyman wrote. "Even should the disease spread to certain European countries, modern sanitation of cities, the knowledge of disinfectants and improved disinfecting appliances, and modern knowledge of the disease itself will doubtless enable it to be confined within reasonable limits." Laboratory work taking place on a far coast done by a man he did not respect enough to utter his name aloud was not going to change Wyman's mind.

With no authority to reimpose a quarantine and no support, Kinyoun forced himself to stay silent on Angel Island and take the abuse. He felt a duty to act, regardless of how the public felt about him, yet he was frustrated by his lack of options. He had come to believe that advances in the science of bacteriology and immunology would soon render all disease a thing of the past, leaving any death from illness that happened under his watch a heavy stone on his conscience. "The infection of innocent persons, in my mind, is nothing more or less than deliberate or premeditated manslaughter," he wrote in a letter to a friend. At best, he hoped that Wong Chut King's death would prove to be an outlier and that the fumigations undertaken during the short-lived quarantine would be enough to prevent a full epidemic. Yet he knew that if the disease continued to spread without a quick response, it would bring the misery now felt in Hong Kong, with its mass graves and abandoned city blocks, to American shores.

While Kinyoun paced his island laboratory, the Sanitation Department continued its inspection of Chinatown, an exercise largely aimed at smothering rumors spreading across the country that San Francisco was teeming with plague. Twenty-five volunteer physicians accompanied by a squad of policemen went door to door, ostensibly on the lookout for cases of serious illness or unsanitary conditions. The men took special care to avoid finding anything incriminating, even in places famous for their filth. The hotel where Wong Chut King died, which was known for the putrid smell resulting from open sewer lines spilling into its subterranean rooms, was found to be "not so inviting as it might be, but the same could be said of basements in all buildings," said Dr. Chalmers, the chief sanitary inspector, after completing his rounds.

Nearly a week had passed since Wong Chut King's death and no further victims were found. The press in San Francisco declared the city safe once more. "The bubonic scare has collapsed," the *Chronicle* proclaimed. Then, as if on cue, the bloated body of Chu Gam, a twenty-two-year-old laborer, was discovered at 723 Sacramento Street, two short blocks from Portsmouth Square.

Chu's remains had evidently sat undisturbed for several days, sending the body into an advanced stage of decomposition. Neighbors did not complain as the smell of death overwhelmed the three-story flophouse where the man had lived, nor did the health inspectors pick up on the stench that was noticeable on the street outside. Only when a local undertaker intervened and attempted to obtain a burial permit did the Health Board become aware of Chu's death. An autopsy was ordered, but the procedure was nearly made impossible by the pungent mix of gas and bloody foam emanating from the corpse, evidence that the internal organs had begun to rupture and decay. Rotting flesh obscured the search for buboes. Nevertheless, a doctor from the Board of Health removed a tissue sample and sent it to Kinyoun, who soon identified the presence of plague bacilli. It was the second death attributed to the disease within a span of eight days.

Others soon followed. The decomposing body of Ng Ach Ging, a thirty-five-year-old Chinese cook, was deposited outside an undertaker's office at 905 Dupont Street two days later. The following afternoon, the body of Lee Sung Kong, aged forty-seven, was found abandoned in a Chinatown alleyway. Kinyoun took part in the autopsies of both men and found clear samples of plague bacilli, a discovery that both confirmed his worst fears and escalated them further. Plague was not only spreading, he realized, but Chinese residents—possibly with the assistance of Western-trained doctors familiar with the methods of bacteriology—appeared to be hiding victim's bodies in hopes that the decomposition process would obscure the true cause of death, turning the survival of the city into a cat-and-mouse game.

Kinyoun still clung to the hope that the rising death toll would shake the city out of its denial, yet he grew more incredulous as the press refused to admit the danger that San Francisco was in. "We do not believe that a single person has ever died of bubonic plague in this city," the *Chronicle* wrote in an editorial after the body of the fourth plague victim was found. "It is useless to say that the bodies have been spirited away. They must be buried and before they can be buried there must be a permit."

It took one of the most powerful men in the country to push the city into action. On Sunday, March 18, twelve days after the discovery of Wong Chut King's body, the *New York Journal*, owned by William Randolph Hearst, published a special national edition that declared "The Black Plague Creeps into America." Oversized drawings of cemeteries and emaciated plague victims shared the front page with articles detailing what the paper described as a growing panic on San Francisco's streets. Hearst, himself born and raised in the city as the only child of a millionaire mining executive, followed up on the publication by personally sending telegrams to the health officers of every major city in the country, warning them to take precautions against the spread of plague from San Francisco.

Almost immediately, ships hailing from the city were quarantined in ports along the Pacific coast. In Victoria, British Columbia, quarantine officers demanded that luggage and clothing belonging to passengers from the city be fumigated and then destroyed; in the tourist destination of Mazatlán, Mexico, passengers on a Pacific Coast Steamship Company ship that had left San Francisco the week before were forced to spend three days in quarantine before landing. Merchants in Alaska, then at the tail end of what was known as the Klondike Gold Rush, began refusing shipments of goods that originated in the San Francisco Bay. Hotels in Denver quickly began to fill, as travelers from cities along the East Coast who had intended to go to San Francisco turned back upon reading the Hearst report and began to mix with those escaping California.

"On the train from 'Frisco I was surprised at the large number with whom I conversed who frankly admitted that they were simply fleeing from the Asiatic plague, which, without any doubt at all, is now found to be in San Francisco," a man from Albany, New York, told a reporter. "It is true there may be only a few cases of the plague, but if there is even one case it is enough to frighten away many tourists who, all their lives, have heard of how deadly this plague is and how rapidly it spreads when introduced into any country . . . On the very train which I came eastward there was represented almost every state east of the Missouri."

As it felt its prospects dim, San Francisco looked for someone to blame, and soon found it in the out-of-town newspapers that were so willing to report the truth of Kinyoun's findings. "There appears to be no motive at all in reading this report other than one of pure deviltry," one merchant told the local press after noticing yet another story detailing the spread of the disease in San Francisco, urging his fellow residents to stop subscribing to any publication that printed stories confirming the presence of plague in the city. The Manufacturers and Producers Association, a trade group representing some of the city's largest employers, called a special meeting at which it adopted a resolution praising the hometown newspapers which "defensed the city against the hurtful story that bubonic plague existed here" and imploring them to continue to "have a care for the general interests of the city" with their coverage. An editorial in the *Call*, meanwhile, opined that the Hearst report was the worst example of the cruel sensationalism of yellow journalism. "The whole business is a piece of idiocy, but, unfortunately for California, as harmful as if there was really occasion for it," the paper wrote. "The man who walks the streets of San Francisco today is as safe from plague as he is in New York or Boston, but after the

Journal's scare edition it will take several months to convince people that this is the truth."

With no other recourse, San Francisco turned to the Board of Health, which its newspapers had long derided, for redemption. Health authorities ordered a more extensive cleanup and inspection of Chinatown—and with it came the chance to discover the full extent of the threat the city now faced. "There is no use evading the issue. The Chinese quarter of this city is infected with plague. The Chinese are concealing the cases, and for this reason the board has increased the corps of inspectors . . . San Francisco is fronted with a serious condition, and the citizens must prepare to meet it," the president of the Board of Health said in an article that ran in the Scripps–McRae chain of newspapers in the Midwest, but his admission received no mention in San Francisco papers.

Sanitation remained a relatively new concept in the United States, where as recently as 1850 Frederick Law Olmsted—now known chiefly as the co-designer of New York's Central Park—had toured the country to highlight everyday acts of filthiness for which he deemed "barbarous too mild a term." In Virginia hotels, he wrote, "every clean towel I got during my stay was a matter of special negotiation"; in Mississippi, the hotel bed he was offered was "furnished with soiled sheets and greasy pillows" used by previous guests. A request for drinking water in Texas resulted in a field hand smashing ice hanging from the side of a building with his hand and pouring the mixture of dirt, water and grime into a mud-streaked glass.

Cities offered filth on a grander scale. New York's first sanitary survey, conducted in 1864, noted overflowing toilets, manure-infested streets, and a persistent stream of blood leaking out of a Midtown slaughterhouse and flowing for two blocks along 39th Street to the river. Pedestrians would pay a nickel to young boys who stood at intersections along Broadway with brooms, ready to sweep a clear path through the slime.

Medicine at the time did not yet fully accept the germ theory of disease—the understanding that microscopic organisms invade and reproduce within host bodies, causing illness. Even sanitary reformers such as Edwin Chadwick remained convinced that filth itself spread disease, despite mounting evidence to the contrary. In 1854, John Snow, physician to Queen Victoria, traced an outbreak of cholera in London to a single contaminated well. Though Snow would later isolate the bacterium that transmitted the disease, Chadwick continued to believe that it was the putrid smell of the water, and not an unseen organism living within it, that spread infection.

Where early sanitarians did agree was on the need to change human behavior. Some of the first public health officers began focusing not only on structural improvements—maintaining clean sources of water and calling for the installation of private toilets in all buildings among them—but on private habits as well, emphasizing the need for daily bathing and teeth cleaning at a time when neither was common. Within a generation, good personal hygiene was considered a mark of Americanness, with newly arrived immigrants of all ethnicities often derided first for their filthy bodies, and later for foreign behaviors that they did not shed.

San Francisco had never organized a sanitation campaign of any significance, leaving Kinyoun skeptical that it could. His misgivings grew as he watched a platoon of seventy-five health inspectors and thirty physicians, each one accompanied by armed policemen, swarm through Chinatown's narrow alleyways as if they were an invading army. Officials pounded on residents' doors and, when refused admission, broke them down with axes and sledgehammers before ransacking apartments. More often than not, the inspection ended with health officials and policemen walking away with any valuables they could find.

Rumors of beatings and rape at the hands of health inspectors spread through Chinatown, cementing fears that the plague cleanup was merely an excuse for violence. Some Chinese women, fearful that the Western physicians conducting the raids were intent on poisoning them, hid their babies during the day and nursed them only in the darkest hours of the night. Unable to live with the embarrassment of a group of armed white men bursting into their homes and ordering them to present their naked groins for inspection, men throughout the district vowed to get even with what the Chinese began calling the "wolf doctors" who preyed upon them. One particularly loathsome official was singled out in an article in the *Chinese Western Daily*, which said that residents of Chinatown would be "glad to bathe in his blood."

Fearing that any violent resistance would give the city a reason to burn down Chinatown and repopulate the district with white residents, the Chinese resorted to deception. One professor at the University of California, Berkeley who volunteered on the cleanup described coming upon a bustling house on Waverly Place in which five Chinese men were seated at a table, apparently playing a game of dominoes. A cursory inspection revealed no obvious cases of infection and the team of doctors continued their rounds. Two hours later, the police received a call from neighbors reporting a death in the same house. The professor returned to the now deserted building to find the dead body of one of the men he had seen just hours before, sitting in the same position. Only then did he realize that the man's roommates had propped the corpse up against the table and pretended to converse with it while the inspectors were there.

The district's open spaces offered little safety. Authorities slathered suspect buildings and streets with toxic chemicals, leaving residents struggling to breathe. Merchants complained that sulfur sprayed indiscriminately by health inspectors ruined their merchandise and made even the healthy feel sick. To protect themselves from the contaminants of a place they neither trusted nor understood, health authorities installed fumigation stations in Portsmouth Square, through which every inspector and policeman was required to pass on their way in and out of the district. Policemen on horseback stood sentry along the borders of Chinatown, scanning the streets for anyone who seemed obviously ill, while inspectors posted at railway stations and along the docks kept watch for Chinese trying to leave the city.

After two weeks of cleanup with no new cases identified, Phelan sent a telegram addressed to the mayors of the fifty largest cities in the Eastern half of the country, promising that Chinatown was now cleaner than at any other time in its history and that all signs of plague were gone. As March turned to April, health inspectors began pulling back from the district, confident that the danger had passed.

The calm would not last the month. On April 24, the body of Law Ann, a thirty-eight-year-old Chinese man who had come to California as a child, was found lying at the end of St. Louis Alley, a dead-end path just off Jackson Street. A dark bubo bulged from his left groin. Kinyoun took a sample of tissue from the body and soon confirmed that the man had died of plague.

Other deaths soon followed. Lim Fa Muey, a sixteen-year-old girl, suddenly collapsed and died on May 11 while working on the floor of a cigar factory, making her the first female victim of the disease. An inspection of her body revealed a walnut-sized bubo on her right thigh that had been covered up with a sticky black plaster, a sign that she had sought treatment from a Chinese healer. The same day, the decomposed body of Chu Sam, a thirty-eight-year-old merchant, was found at 717 Jackson Street. Its degraded condition rendered a formal autopsy impossible, yet tissue samples revealed plague bacilli. Chin Moon, a sixteen-year-old girl working as a servant for a Chinese family residing at 730 Commercial Street, died in the Pacific Hospital on May 15 after complaining of headaches, high fever and pain in the right thigh. Western physicians practicing in Chinatown initially diagnosed typhoid fever, before Kinyoun's examination of tissue samples from the body uncovered plague. On May 17, Herr Woon Jock, a fifty-three-year-old Chinese laborer who had recently arrived in the city from Stockton, died at 740 Pacific Street, and an autopsy showed a swelling bubo on his left thigh.

Within the span of one week, the death toll from the disease had jumped to eight confirmed victims. Kinyoun suspected that dozens more had simply vanished, never to become a part of the official record nor give him any clue of where the disease was heading next. "How many Chinamen have died from plague and how many corpses of victims from this disease awaited shipment to China no white man will ever know," he wrote in a letter to a friend in Washington.

Kinyoun spent frantic hours retracing the last days of each victim's life, trying to find any shared connections that would have allowed plague to spread from one host to another. Yet he found nothing. The nearest victims had lived two blocks away from each other, but did not frequent the same stores or restaurants, while the furthest apart appeared never to have come within eight blocks of one another. With no linked source of infection, there could only be one conclusion: an epidemic was at hand.

Kinyoun rushed off a telegram directly to Wyman in Washington, not bothering to go through the usual middlemen who served as a buffer between them: "Examination plague suspect completed. Diagnosis confirmed by bacteriological examination. No connection traced to first at present. Don't give this information to public. Will write reasons for secrecy." The next day, he followed with a longer telegram which revealed his increasing desperation. "As requested, secrecy required first case on account of vicious attacks [by] local press," he wrote. "Regard situation very serious; will require almost superhuman efforts to control now, so much time has been lost. Over 35,000 people must be controlled."

He saw but one solution: the widespread administration of a still-experimental vaccine among the Chinese in the city, even if the procedure had to be done by force. Developed by Waldemar Mordecai Haffkine, a Ukrainian scientist who, like Kinyoun, had once studied with Louis Pasteur, the so-called Haffkine serum had been developed by growing plague cells taken from cadavers and subjecting them to high heat in order to kill their ability to multiply. After potential patients in several villages refused to receive any serum that included plague germs, the first tests had been conducted on a group of prisoners in Bombay three years before. The serum was shown to reduce the risk of infection by half.

Yet its side effects—high fever, violent vomiting, and a deep but temporary reddening of the skin—would leave its recipients incapacitated for two days at least, and required additional injections every six months to remain effective. "Inoculation, although its results are extremely important and promising, is a prophylactic rather than a treatment, a wall against the enemy rather than a weapon with which to meet it," noted an early report on the serum's effectiveness which ran in the well-read journal *Public Health Reports*. Kinyoun estimated that it would cost at least $100,000—a sum equivalent to $2.7 million today—to buy and administer enough doses of the serum to cover everyone living in Chinatown. The high cost was warranted, he urged Wyman. "If depopulation should be necessary, ten times this amount will be required," he warned.

Wyman agreed and immediately shipped twenty thousand doses of the Haffkine serum to San Francisco, with the promise of additional supplies once they became available. Despite the turbulent history between the men, Wyman now found himself forced to rely on and trust Kinyoun as his surrogate in a moment of crisis. He attempted to flatter Kinyoun with responsibility, sending him a personal telegram in which he admitted that in the fight ahead he would have to function as the "one man in supreme charge" of all efforts to stop the disease from destroying San Francisco. Successfully breaking the epidemic would require cordoning off Chinatown and instituting house-to-house inspections, all while preventing any Chinese from leaving the city on its ferries or rails—a job that only a man with Kinyoun's experience could handle, Wyman suggested.

While he hoped that the abundance of praise would have its intended effect, Wyman never lost sight of the fact that such a plan would require a sense of tact that Kinyoun lacked even on his best days. Without telling Kinyoun, Wyman sent direct telegrams to the Chinese consul general in San Francisco, pleading with him to "have the Chinese comply cheerfully with necessary measures" and to contact the Surgeon General's office in Washington at once should matters get out of hand.

As he waited for the shipments of the Haffkine serum to arrive, Kinyoun met privately with Mayor Phelan, members of the Board of Health and the heads of the Merchants Association in a closed room at City Hall, and impressed upon them the danger that they all now faced. The men badgered Kinyoun with questions for nearly eight straight hours, determined to find inconsistencies in his assessment of the threat. Unable to do so, they eventually conceded and offered their support should Kinyoun insist on a prolonged closure of Chinatown, though it would mean sacrificing a lucrative summer's worth of trade. Their main concern, however, was the "earnest desire that no newspaper or other publicity be made, for obvious reasons" until the plan was set in motion, an aide who accompanied Kinyoun to the meeting wrote in a private telegram to Wyman that night.

Though he now had support, Kinyoun saw only risks ahead. The city's inaction after Wong Chut King's death had allowed the plague to become entrenched in a small but densely populated portion of the city; any harsh measures that might scare those living in the plague zone into fleeing outside the district would potentially expand the grip of the disease further. A "great danger lies in fact of [an] exodus which [will] necessarily occur as soon as house to house inspection begins," he cautioned Wyman. In response, Wyman reassigned Marine Health Service inspectors to guard train stations in Reno and at points along the Oregon border with orders to detain and question any Chinese passengers they encountered, forming a makeshift wall intended to pen the plague within California.

It soon became clear that residents might flee the neighborhood before Kinyoun had an opportunity to seal them in. In Hawaii, health officials had inoculated thousands of Chinese with the Haffkine serum without complaint. Yet coming at a time when distrust of compulsory smallpox vaccinations spurred Americans of all ethnicities to pull their children from public schools, most Chinese in San Francisco saw the Haffkine serum as ineffective at best and suspected that it was actually a plan to poison them. Tongs threatened to harm anyone who submitted to the vaccine, prompting Ng Poon Chew, the editor of the influential Chinese-language newspaper *Chinese Western Daily*, to publicly receive a dose in hopes of setting a positive example to others. A mob soon surrounded his building on Sacramento Street, forcing him to hide in Oakland for several days, and his newspaper immediately lost half of its subscribers. Days later, Ng came out of hiding and broke ranks with other powerful Chinese who supported the inoculation drive, declaring vaccination a form of modern torture.

It was a sentiment shared widely throughout the city, regardless of race. Doctors had never been trusted in San Francisco, and the idea of voluntarily receiving an injection of dead plague germs sounded suicidal at a time when diseases such as tuberculosis and typhoid fever routinely killed men and women in their prime. For all of his technical brilliance, Kinyoun still had much to learn about life outside the laboratory, and he failed to understand why he would need to go to Chinatown himself and explain how and why the serum could save lives. Once again unable to forge a human connection that would make his medical understanding truly useful, he could only watch as men with no scientific skill or understanding shaped public opinion against him. J. A. Boyle, a reporter for the *San Francisco Examiner*, submitted to a dose of the Haffkine serum to show its side effects. The resulting article described shooting pains in his neck and head, a partial paralysis of his arm, and a high fever that left him "drifting into stupor," and solidified public opposition to the vaccine.

"Residents of San Francisco are being advised to resist by certain whites," Kinyoun wrote in a telegram to Wyman in the following days. Refusing to bend, Kinyoun sent health inspectors with doses of the Haffkine serum door to door in Chinatown, a move which the Chinese saw as a provocation. Pamphlets written in Chinese appeared throughout the district, repeating the tongs' warnings against submitting to the injections. More than seven hundred Chinatown residents joined in protests in front of the Chinese consulate building, angry at the escalation of a plan they saw as tantamount to murder and destroyed several windows before police ordered them to disperse.

At the request of Chinese officials, Kinyoun traveled to the consulate building the following day, where he found several high-ranking officers of the Chinese Six Companies waiting for him. It was the first time that Kinyoun had met with the men in person, whom he regarded with an odd mixture of admiration and bigotry. For all of his achievements in understanding the human body at a cellular level, he was never quite capable of ignoring the outer shell of race. The men of the Chinese Six Companies "rule with a rod of iron and are as autocratic as the Empress of China," Kinyoun later wrote in a letter to a friend. "They are men of superior intelligence when compared to those of their race, possessing the shrewdness, coupled together with all the other disagreeable features of the Chinese character, which makes them an enemy not to be despised."

If it continued, the vaccination campaign would lead to a full riot that might spill beyond Chinatown, officers of the Chinese Six Companies told Kinyoun, and implored him to call it off. With Wyman's reminders to control his temper no doubt ringing in his head, Kinyoun replied that the choice whether to receive the serum remained voluntary. But if the plague scare was not dealt with now, there would likely be harsher measures coming in the future that he could not control, he warned. At that moment, aides burst into the room and announced that over a thousand Chinese residents had surrounded the consulate and were throwing rocks at its windows, inflamed by Kinyoun's presence inside. Only after an escort of police officers arrived was Kinyoun able to escape and make his way back to Angel Island.

No one in Chinatown submitted to the Haffkine serum over the following three days, deflating what little hope Kinyoun still harbored. The discovery of another badly decomposed body and suspected plague case further unnerved him. Though he had no confirmation, he grew convinced that the worst of his fears were being realized. "Exodus has begun," he wrote in a telegram to Wyman. Fearing what he perceived to be Kinyoun's tendency to panic, Wyman immediately wired back. Keeping his tone neutral so as not to push Kinyoun over the edge, "Advise that you use tact and discretion in enforcing Haffkine inoculation of Chinese and be not too precipitate or harsh. End will be more certainly and easily gained . . . it is suggested here that it would materially influence the Chinese if some whites were vaccinated," he counseled.

With no allies, no sense of diplomacy and no natural authority, Kinyoun found no white San Franciscans who would agree to serve as an example of the serum's safety and had to call off his plans. Residents of the city, no matter their race, seemed to exhibit no fear of the disease, nor any sense of urgency that they were in its path. The apparent comfort with ignoring Kinyoun's warnings dispelled the worries of tourists who had been hesitant to visit the city following the reports of plague. The city's population continued to grow and its hotels remained full, filling its streets with people who had no idea of the danger they were in. "People here absolutely in [the] dark as to correct situation, on account of local papers refusing publishing any matter pertaining to epidemic," Kinyoun wired Wyman. Seven days after the start of the drive that he had hoped would protect the city, he could count only 53 Chinese residents who submitted to the vaccination, and 764 San Franciscans overall. With no progress to show for it, an inoculation campaign that could have offered some measure of protection was abandoned, leaving San Francisco no safer than before.

As San Francisco refused to take steps to save itself from the disease, Wyman shifted his focus to preventing plague from spreading across the nation. Bolstered by the Service's federally mandated authority to take all steps necessary to prevent serious diseases from crossing state lines, he directed agents to inspect all trains and ships before they were permitted to leave California and detain any Chinese or Japanese passengers regardless of their health. It was in effect a racial quarantine, aimed at preventing all Asian residents of California— who were already suspect because of the color of their skin—from carrying plague eastward. Wyman submitted the proposal to President William McKinley on May 21, 1900, and received his approval the same day. Marine Hospital Service inspectors moved into position, slowing all interstate traffic leaving California until they could ensure that no Asians were on board.

Three days later, several powerful law firms in San Francisco joined in a lawsuit filed in the U.S. Circuit Court of Northern California. The plaintiff was a Chinese merchant by the name of Wong Wai, who demanded an injunction that would prevent any restraint of the free movement of Chinese residents at a time when the existence of plague had not been officially declared. Kinyoun, along with all members of the city's Board of Health, was named as a defendant, though he did not attend the trial. His attention was diverted instead by an anonymous threat warning him that the Marine Hospital Service's overnight patrol boats would soon be run down and destroyed by Chinese tongs.

As the court proceedings began, Kinyoun was holed up on Angel Island, sending urgent telegrams to the Secretary of the Navy requesting warships and patrols to prevent San Francisco's Asian population from escaping across the bay under cover of night. After four days of hearings, Judge William Morrow released a decision that made Kinyoun's requests moot. While laudatory in intent, the plague prevention measures "directed against the Asiatic or Mongolian race as a class, without regard to the previous condition, habits, exposure to disease, or residence of the individual" were clear violations of those people's constitutional rights, Morrow wrote. He issued a restraining order preventing Kinyoun or any of his agents from interfering in any way with the Chinese residents of San Francisco. Kinyoun was despondent. "Under decision, believe situation to United States very grave," he wired Wyman. "The decision is far-reaching, and practically nullifies all acts of Federal Government within state, as well as preventing cooperation, aid, and assistance . . . [it is] the most serious blow Service has received since assuming quarantine measures."

Businessmen clad in dark suits and bowler hats crammed into a sweltering ballroom the following day, called there by the powerful state Board of Health for what it would only say was an urgent matter. In the center of the room sat representatives of the Southern Pacific Company, whose rails heading eastward remained the lifeblood of the state. No one wanted to be the first to speak, knowing that the future of the state hung on their words. Kinyoun stood to the side, waiting for his chance to make allies among the members of the board—the only doctors in the state whose regulatory authority rivaled his own.

Only after the room was full and the doors were shut did a state health official reveal the reason for the meeting: Texas and Louisiana were both considering a quarantine of all people and goods originating from California. If there was no definite way to show that the plague was contained, other states were sure to follow. It went unsaid that any such declaration could ruin California's economy for a generation, leaving the Golden State unable to shed its association with disease. Dr. W. F. Blunt, the chief health officer of Texas, took the stage and said that he was especially unnerved by what he saw as the open mingling of Chinese and white residents on the streets of San Francisco, a situation that would only end in the spread of what he saw as an "Asiatic" disease to the white population. Perhaps, Blunt suggested, if the Chinese were segregated into one district, then he might consider keeping the borders of Texas open to California.

Judge Morrow's ruling the day before had rendered the Marine Hospital Service powerless to implement such a plan. The only thing left, it seemed, was for the state Board of Health—unmentioned in the federal court's decision—to impose a full and indefinite quarantine of Chinatown, cordoning everyone who lived inside regardless of their race. It would undeniably cause economic pain, yet that would be nothing compared with the permanent stigma that would come if other states refused free entry to anyone or anything connected with California.

Dr. D. D. Crowley, the acting president of the state Board of Health, called upon Kinyoun to address the meeting, introducing him as "second to none as a bacteriologist." Kinyoun rose to the stage and agreed that quarantine appeared to be the sole option remaining. Plague was here, he warned the men before him, and they were the only people powerful enough to stop it. The room fell silent as the weight of Kinyoun's words sank in.

"At the present time, Dr. Kinyoun, you are powerless," said Dr. Crowley at last.

"I have no power except to talk," Kinyoun replied, straining to keep the panic out of his voice.

CHAPTER 6

QUARANTINE

The morning quiet was punctured by the sound of a hundred policemen moving into position. They formed a perimeter around Chinatown, preventing any escape. Additional officers stepped forward carrying planks of wood, cement blocks and coils of barbed wire. As residents looked on, the men began building an eight-foot-high fence along the borders of the district. Barbed wire was bunched along the top and the approaches to the barrier, its sharp points glimmering like the thorns of overgrown bushes. By noon, more than ten thousand people were sealed within the new quarantine zone, unsure if they would ever again be free. All streetcar lines running through the district were stopped and all shipments of food across the line refused, once again marooning the Chinese in the city. Chinatown residents were now like "fish caught in a net," in the words of the *Chinese Western Daily*.

Desperate, hungry and unable to reach their jobs outside the quarantine area, more than a thousand Chinese surrounded the headquarters of the Chinese Six Companies demanding action. While Chinese leaders filed injunctions in the local federal court and the Chinese minister in Washington lodged an official complaint with Secretary of State John Hay, ad hoc vigilance committees formed on the streets, aimed at punishing anyone cooperating with the Western physicians who seemed intent on setting Chinatown ablaze. The Chinese would "rather die than have our town burned," one Chinese man told reporters.

A mob surrounded an undertaker by the name of Wing Tie as he led a horse carting three wooden coffins near the quarantine line, convinced that the sight of a man wheeling caskets would inflame the suspicions of health authorities who believed the Chinese were concealing illness. The mob hurled the empty coffins into the street and then pelted Wing Tie's store with rocks, shattering its glass and sending the man into hiding. Rumors that health authorities were administering forced vaccinations brought hundreds of angry men into Portsmouth Square, where they clashed with police brandishing clubs. Unable to break through the quarantine lines, the bloodied crowd moved on toward Waverly Place, where they tore up cobblestones from the street and attacked the store of a man said to be secretly feeding information to Western doctors, leaving it in ruins.

As Chinatown edged closer to anarchy, Kinyoun prepared for what he now believed was the only way to ensure that the plague epidemic did not kill millions: removing every Asian resident from San Francisco and into temporary custody, by force if necessary. Identifying living patients carrying the disease within the quarantine zone was an "impossible task," he telegrammed Wyman, given the lack of trust between the Chinese and city officials. "Inspectors have not found a sick person, nor can they discover the dead; these are found in undertaker's shops, discovered by other persons," he wrote.

More than a thousand Chinese and Japanese who lived outside the quarantine zone had fled to other parts of the state as soon as the wall went up, exacerbating Kinyoun's fear that carriers of the disease were already on the move. After securing funding from the state Board of Health and approval from Wyman and the Secretary of War in Washington, Kinyoun rented several warehouses on Mission Rock— a small, gravel-strewn island at the mouth of Mission Bay—for use as temporary barracks to house the city's Asian population until Chinatown was disinfected and its buildings demolished. Should the warehouses not be large enough to hold the more than ten thousand residents of Chinatown, he sketched a layout for a tent city on the opposite end of Angel Island, far enough away that he would not have to worry about the disease spreading to the sprawling Marine Hospital Service station. He knew that military assistance would be required to force the Chinese into submission, but he believed it was the only way it might be possible to contain the disease.

While consumed in planning, Kinyoun received an unannounced visit from the president of the Chamber of Commerce, who requested a private meeting in his office at Angel Island. Once out of earshot of aides, the man offered what Kinyoun would later describe as "large and handsome presents" in exchange for declaring the city free of plague. Kinyoun refused the bribe on the spot. That the man felt comfortable offering him a payoff despite his central role in implementing the quarantine and a public reputation for prudishness only confirmed Kinyoun's suspicions that other doctors in the city were regularly putting money before duty and knowingly attributing plague deaths to other illnesses. He had long disliked daily life in California, from the taste of the fish that his sons caught at the small pier outside their barrack at Angel Island to the way that a golden glimmer of opportunity seemed to blind its citizens to any morals that stood in their way. Now, for the first time, he realized that his distaste had devolved into disgust, and he hardened his resolve to protect the country from a place he believed was wicked to its core.

"It appears that the 'commercial interests' of San Francisco are more dear to the inhabitants than the preservation of human life," he wrote in a long letter to a friend in Washington. "No sentiment has been expressed against a possible danger arising to the people, to their wives and children. These people seem perfectly indifferent, whether or not bubonic plague exists in San Francisco, so long as they can sell their products and make large percentages on their investments . . . It would be difficult to say what will be necessary to awaken this people to their responsibility as citizens of the United States, and to the fact that California is a part of the Union. The prevailing sentiment here is that California is still a republic; that the 'Bear' is above the Stars and Stripes; and that the 'native son' takes precedence over the citizen. The presence of the United States is tolerated simply for the sake of convenience, and for what material benefits that can derive therefrom. In the matter of pure patriotism I believe it exists here in less quantity and poorer quality, than can be found in any place in the United States."

As the possibility of bloodshed bubbled higher in Chinatown, Kinyoun received a telegram from Wyman, a man he increasingly saw as too afraid to travel out west and put himself on the line. Such timidity on the part of a man who was supposed to be a leader gnawed at Kinyoun, inflaming his natural tendency to ignore anyone he did not respect. Still, he followed orders, not yet desperate enough to risk open insubordination. Wyman alerted Kinyoun to the fact that Dr. George F. Shrady, who had become one of the nation's most prominent doctors after attending to President Ulysses S. Grant during his final hours, was then secretly en route to San Francisco. Once there, he would investigate the bubonic plague scare and write a series of articles confirming or denying the presence of the disease that would be published simultaneously in the *New York Herald* and the *San Francisco Call*. Kinyoun was to meet with Shrady as soon as he reached San Francisco and assist him in any way possible.

Though Kinyoun welcomed the idea of finally working with someone who respected his East Coast credentials, he knew that nothing with Shrady would be easy. He had met him once before, while serving on cholera duty in New York City, and came away unimpressed. The man was a famous windbag, more accustomed to delivering lectures in front of admiring audiences than working in a laboratory or treating patients. He had let his Civil War accolades and deep lineage, which included both grandfathers having taken up arms on the side of the colonies during the American Revolution, get to his head, and he now carried himself with a pomposity bordering on the ridiculous. Kinyoun suspected that Shrady would not even know what bubonic plague looked like under a microscope, yet sought him out as directed.

It took several days after Shrady arrived in the city for Kinyoun to gain admittance into what he would later sarcastically refer to as "the presence." Shrady had transformed a suite in the Palace Hotel into a miniature version of the newsroom of the *New York Herald*, with news clerks stationed in front of typewriters on makeshift desks, and was preparing for his first tour of Chinatown the following day when Kinyoun arrived. Kinyoun listened as Shrady began a monologue about what he expected to see and how his readers would react. Kinyoun interrupted him to say that "until this time it had not been possible for anyone to have anything published in the San Francisco press that in any way reflected the true condition of affairs," a condition that "practically meant the suppression of news," he would later write. Shrady responded that he had the authority to publish whatever he wished and relaunched into his sermon, focusing this time on how readers would be thrilled to learn that he was in town.

The more the man talked, the more Kinyoun realized that Shrady's plan was to say that no true cases of plague had been found before he arrived in the city and then discover infected patients himself, making him a national hero once more. His accolades assured, Shrady would then go on to call for the total and immediate destruction of Chinatown by fire and dynamite. Envisioning the riots that would ensue if Shrady's plans were made known, Kinyoun "begged him by everything holy never to advocate such a thing as that at the present time, unless he had ten thousand troops at his back," he later wrote in a letter to a friend. Shrady seemed uninterested in Kinyoun's warnings and the meeting soon ended.

All of San Francisco waited over the following days for Shrady's verdict. "The people of San Francisco have reason for the deepest congratulations. One of the most expert bacteriologists in the world and a physician famed for his ability is in the city at the instance of the *New York Herald* and the *Call,* to make a thorough and absolutely impartial investigation of the facts which have led to the sensational reports that bubonic plague is in this city," the *Call* reported in a front-page spread. Shrady's fame was so great that his dispatches in the *Call* were reprinted in part in competing papers, something unheard of at a time when editorial pages delighted in mocking their adversaries.

In his first article, Shrady detailed a daytime journey into Chinatown and to the Globe Hotel, where Wong Chut King, the first known victim of the disease, had lived. As he walked along the streets of the district accompanied by a police officer, Shrady grew unnerved by "a smothered firing of vengeance in the expression of almost every Chinaman you would meet. This was decidedly notable and made one feel most uncomfortable," he wrote. Only after an officer subtly informed him that he carried a gun under his overcoat did Shrady begin to feel at ease. He descended into the subterranean passages beneath the Globe Hotel, holding three candles ahead of him to light the way along a path that was "twisted, uneven, low, dark, dirty and in every way forbidding, with smell intolerable." He attempted to enter the apartments of the building's residents, evidently in hopes of finding a living person carrying the disease, but was rebuffed at every turn. He made no attempt to understand why, finding fault in those in whom he saw only filth. The Chinese "seemed to have a superstitious idea that the white man is a natural enemy, even after death. Often when an inspection of a suspected house was attempted the doors would be locked because of the apparent stupidity of the occupants . . . In fact, it was quite a frequent occurrence during an active house to house inspection for the Chinese to take their sick over the roofs of their house and thus deceive the inspector," he wrote.

Shrady failed to uncover any evidence of plague, a fact that the *Call* highlighted in a separate front-page article that ran along his first-person dispatch. Kinyoun, sensing an opportunity, brought a package containing cells from nine confirmed plague cases and his own microscope to the doctor's hotel room the following day. With Shrady uncharacteristically quiet, Kinyoun detailed the case histories of each victim, and then gave Shrady a tutorial in how the disease presented itself in the body and how to identify it via microscope and grow it in a culture. The next morning, he asked Shrady to accompany him to the autopsy of a suspected plague case at a Chinatown morgue, certain that the doctor could not pass up an opportunity which would allow him to personally announce the discovery of a plague victim to the nation.

Spectators watching marching bands performing in a Decoration Day parade—the precursor of the modern Memorial Day—clogged the streets as the men made their way toward Chinatown and the quarantine line. Once inside the district, policemen protected them as they walked to 706 Pacific Street, where a body lay waiting in a coffin shop. Dozens of Chinese were standing outside the building and dozens more trailed the doctors in a quiet procession, all waiting to hear the results of the autopsy. Kinyoun and Shrady stepped inside the funeral home and found the body of Dang Hong, a forty-year-old man who had died after complaining of a venereal disease, lying under a dirty sheet. The body was in good condition and exhibited few obvious signs of plague. No buboes were present, and no swelling was evident in the lymph nodes in the groin or armpits. Nevertheless, Kinyoun took a sample of tissue from the inguinal gland, located near the pelvis, and prepared a slide. He and Shrady each took a turn examining it under a microscope, and agreed that it appeared to be plague. Kinyoun then took additional tissue samples from the body for use in animal inoculations, which would confirm the diagnosis.

"It is with the greatest regret that this statement must be made, but the plain truth must be told," Shrady wrote the following day in a front-page article. "This, as I understand it, is what the public has asked for. Now the time has come to face the issue calmly, deliberately and judiciously." Plague was indeed in San Francisco, and the city must respond. He counseled the mayor to take no drastic actions, and its residents not to flee. There had yet to be a person with the disease found alive, he noted, and there were no signs of an epidemic that could reach beyond the quarantine line. And though the disease was now confirmed, that did not necessarily mean that all of San Francisco was in danger. Race, he declared, continued to matter more than plague cells. "The disease is not apt to spread rapidly at first," he wrote. "We must remark also in this connection that it has a special predilection for the Asiatic race and exceptionally attacks the whites."

Though Shrady's series of articles was set to run for another three days, Kinyoun allowed himself to feel hope again. He did not share Shrady's confidence that the disease would naturally confine itself to the city's Asian population, but that was not what mattered at that moment. For the first time in months, a San Francisco paper had printed an article that openly acknowledged that plague was within the city. He quickly issued orders that he knew would have been blocked before Shrady's confirmation of plague. He directed quarantine officers at Angel Island to refuse clean bills of health to outward-bound steamers, an implicit admission that San Francisco was an infected port, and sent letters to the members of the state Board of Health, directing them to prepare quarantine officers to once again patrol the state's borders and prevent any Asians from leaving.

Kinyoun clung to his optimism even as Shrady seemed to back away from the truth of the plague's existence in the city in his article the following morning. While Kinyoun worked to contain the disease, Shrady had participated in the autopsy of a child the day before. With no understanding that Chinese tradition held that the procedure could prevent a person's ascension into the afterlife, he could only gaze with bewilderment when the boy's father had to be restrained by police officers while doctors began the procedure.

No plague bacilli were found in the child's body, leaving Shrady to question whether the disease was truly entrenched in the city. "It might also be said that the plague is not here. Where is it?" he wrote, remarking once again upon the fact that no living person had been found carrying the disease.

The real issue, he held, was the fact that "Chinatown is so notoriously filthy that almost any superlative could fit such a condition." Had the disease been found in New York City, it would have already been wiped out by its superior Board of Sanitation, he boasted. San Francisco was now in its infancy in terms of hygiene and public health, and it was unfair to judge it by diseases that would no doubt be expunged once a sustained cleanup was underway. The city "has never been waked before on sanitary questions as she is now, and there are earnest men here that are backing a movement for reform which may astonish everyone who is awaiting results," he wrote. "So I think it is perfectly warranted on the part of all concerned, here and elsewhere, to say that the real situation is not by any means so bad as it might otherwise be."

Kinyoun requested a meeting with Shrady to learn what was behind his sudden change in opinion, but was refused. He did not know that before the article ran, Shrady had spent hours in the company of Governor Henry Gage, a bombastic man who took personally any perceived slight against the state. A former sheep dealer who had opened a law practice in Los Angeles, Gage rose to prominence by representing the powerful Southern Pacific Railroad. His tenacity gained him favor with the company, which eventually helped guide him into the governor's office. Now, as he walked the corridors of power in the state capital, he went to great lengths to remind everyone he encountered of his rough past. He sported an enormous walrus mustache and made it known that he stowed a Bowie knife in his ever-present cowboy boots. The measures had the intended effect, granting Gage a reputation for churlishness, but the energy he put into the effort left the lingering impression that it was all a show to distract from his inability to govern.

After his election, both Democrats and members of his own party accused Gage of being a pawn for the railroad, and the governor, unused to confrontations that he did not choose, could not recover. By the second year of his administration, he was widely disliked by voters and ostracized by fellow lawmakers. When he received a telegram from John Hay, the U.S. Secretary of State, inquiring into the persistent rumors of plague in San Francisco, he sensed both a danger to California's economy and a welcome distraction from the questions over his fitness for office. His chief asset had always been his willingness to bully, flatter or lie to get his way, and he now turned those skills on a man unused to being treated with anything but deference.

Over dinner at the Cliff House, an elegant eight-story French chateau perched on the rocks above the Pacific Ocean, and later in the doctor's suite at the Palace Hotel, Gage alternated between charming and challenging Shrady. Wasn't it true, Gage asked, that all of the so-called plague bacilli that Shrady inspected had been furnished to him by either Kinyoun or the state Board of Health, and that he had never personally taken a sample of tissue that exhibited signs of the disease? How did he know that the plague tissue he was inspecting hadn't been imported from India or Japan, or been reused from the same patient? And, if he truly believed that he would be exposed to plague upon coming to San Francisco, why hadn't Shrady opted to receive a dose of the Haffkine serum himself? California's fruit crop alone would be worth $25 million that year and would have to be thrown out if other states suspected that plague was within San Francisco, Gage said; wasn't that an awful lot of money to sacrifice for something that Shrady couldn't be sure of?

Shrady shrank under the questioning, unable to find the self-regard that was his constant companion. Within two days of dining with Gage, he repudiated his earlier statement that plague was present in San Francisco. He could no longer be sure that the plague bacilli he had inspected that week had come from a person who died in San Francisco, he wrote, subtly suggesting that Kinyoun and other doctors had conspired to trick him. His confidence in his own eyes gone, he now saw no reason why Chinatown should be quarantined and mocked the idea that plague could pose a danger to the city even if it were there. "It is like quarantining a 10,000 acre field to stop the spread of a little prairie fire in the middle," Shrady wrote. As he prepared to board a train back to New York, Shrady told reporters that he had promised the governor that if there were no new genuine cases of plague by the time he reached the East Coast, then he would publicly recommend that the quarantine be lifted and that the health officials he had worked with be reassigned.

Though betrayed once more, Kinyoun felt only envy as Shrady's train chugged out of view. It was Shrady, and not him, who was heading back to the East Coast with his reputation intact. Kinyoun, meanwhile, continued to shoulder the responsibility of saving millions of lives in a place that cared nothing for him. Given the rare opportunity to tell San Francisco the truth about the danger it faced, Shrady had instead "fallen into the hands of the Philistines," Kinyoun complained in a bitter letter to a friend.

Gage was not finished. He had built his identity around the notion that he was an embodiment of the lost old ways of California, when white ranchers relied on their common sense and brawn to survive, and he resented the incursion of bespectacled doctors from a far coast who had the power to upend everything he had worked for in his life. He called an emergency meeting of the state Board of Health and spent the session upbraiding its members for not performing their own studies on alleged plague victims and relying instead on the opinions of untrustworthy federal health authorities such as Kinyoun. When a doctor challenged him on his medical knowledge, Gage grew furious. He vowed to prevent the state from spending an additional dollar on maintaining the quarantine and to stop the state Board of Health from sharing any information about the cleanup campaign with other states. As further proof that he did not believe that plague posed any danger, he telegraphed his family in Los Angeles and ordered them to come to San Francisco at once.

The governor sent an official response to Secretary Hay in Washington in which he enclosed a fifteen-point letter signed by prominent figures including Levi Strauss and the president of Cooper Medical College that detailed what he called the "plague fake." He pointed to Kinyoun as its chief conspirator. "The medical gentlemen and experts of the City Board of Health and the federal quarantine officer who have ventured the injurious opinions which have spread broadcast over the world the rumor of the existence of the dreadful plague in this great and healthful city of San Francisco have never seen a living case of plague," he wrote. Privately he met with attorneys working for the Chinese Six Companies and offered lines of attack, as they prepared for a hearing before a federal judge to challenge the quarantine.

The proceedings took place before the same Judge Morrow who had halted the previous quarantine weeks before. The Chinese Six Companies presented witnesses who testified that the quarantine line had been obviously gerrymandered to exclude white-occupied buildings, leaving it a racially—rather than medically—segregated zone. Yet the thrust of its case turned instead to the inability of Kinyoun and other Marine Hospital Service doctors to identify a living person suffering from plague. "Dr. Kinyoun, surgeon of the Marine Hospital Service and Quarantine Office of the port of San Francisco, has injected himself into this case as they inject virus into a rat. Did he ever see the plague in Honolulu, Sydney, or India?" asked J. C. Campbell, an attorney for the Six Companies, in his opening statement. While Kinyoun proudly displayed an M.D. "that flourishes as a tail to [his] name, there is nothing to show this Court that [he is a] physician," Campbell charged. A real doctor was someone who practiced with patients, not microscopes. Bacteriology was nothing but a sham, and the bacteriologists who practiced it were emasculated men who, Campbell suggested, could do no better than stay alone in a room with test tubes all day. "The best evidence that plague does not exist here is the fact that the beardless boys who have been playing with these so-called germs are still alive," he said. "They have had injected rats and animals of all descriptions running around their laboratories and escaped uninjured . . . If there has been plague in San Francisco than the Almighty has wrought a miracle to save them for the fire they have tried so hard to kindle."

As he watched the federal government's attorney sputter, Kinyoun felt his last reserves of hope slip away. He sent a telegram to Wyman asking for permission to enact a little-used power that gave the Marine Hospital Service vast sway over interstate travel should Morrow rule against them. Kinyoun knew that, in theory, his agency could prevent entry into a state to anyone who did not carry a certificate of clean health signed by a federal health officer, though the agency had rarely executed that power and it had never been attempted on a scale so enormous. Instead of quarantining just those living in Chinatown, Kinyoun was proposing that the Marine Hospital Service block every person in the state, regardless of ethnicity, from leaving California. "Believe this is the only course now left open since executive of California has seen fit to make misleading statements to State Department concerning conditions here," Kinyoun wrote.

When Wyman did not immediately reply, Kinyoun began laying the groundwork on his own. He had not forgiven Wyman for sending him to Angel Island, and he could not trust a man who refused to travel to San Francisco himself to show the strength to do what was necessary. With his last chance of preventing the disease from spreading eastward at hand, Kinyoun relied solely on the opinion that had always meant the most to him: his own. Unafraid of the repercussions, he ordered Marine Health Service officials to man posts at every railroad crossing along the state's borders and told them to prepare to enact an almost total closure of California.

"A new word has been coined in the parlance of Western language, and that is 'Kinyounism,'" he wrote in a defiant letter to a friend. "Kinyounism is meant to be that a man will carry out his orders irrespective of the wish of the local people; that he will tell the truth whether it is politic to do so or not; that he cannot be bribed, coerced, or jollied into suppressing the truth, particularly to his superiors. I suppose that the word 'Kinyounism' will remain for quite a number of years as one of the set phrases in describing this condition. I hope so at least."

As expected, Judge Morrow declared the sixteen-day quarantine of Chinatown unconstitutional, ruling that the Board of Health had acted "with an evil eye and unequal hand" in drawing borders based primarily on race. Within hours, workers began dismantling the fences around Chinatown. Wagons full of fresh fruit and supplies entered the district for the first time in more than two weeks, ending a siege that had caused some residents to fear starvation.

As he watched the people of Chinatown move freely throughout the city, potentially spreading their germs onto trains and boats and sidewalks, Kinyoun determined that he had run out of options. Every person in the district must be considered a carrier of the disease, and there was nothing stopping any one of them from getting on an eastbound train and spreading death nationwide.

Nothing, except for him.

CHAPTER 7

OUST THE FAKER

At seven o'clock on the morning of June 16, 1900, Kinyoun ordered every railroad and steamship company in San Francisco to stop selling tickets to people heading out of state unless they could produce a certificate that verified their good health signed by himself or another Marine Hospital Service officer. Passengers bound for destinations outside California would from now on first need to head to the upper floor of the north wing of the Ferry Building, where Kinyoun had posted rows of clerks ready to perform cursory examinations that asked for little more than a traveler's name, age and place of birth.

Kinyoun stood in his full uniform and watched as would-be passengers lined up for inspection, the morning sun glinting off the ceremonial sword dangling from his hip. Nearly all whisked through the process without delay. Kinyoun intervened only when several Chinese residents appeared in line, and requested certificates for travel. After going through a detailed health history with each person, Kinyoun rejected their applications on the basis that they had not received a Haffkine injection. Over the course of the day, no white passengers—the vast majority of whom were also unvaccinated—were denied the paperwork that allowed them to board trains and vessels headed out of the state.

Kinyoun posted agents at railroad crossings including Truckee—on the Nevada state line—Ashland, Oregon, and Blake and Yuma, in Arizona, to detain passengers from San Francisco who did not possess a signed health record. He planned to establish internment camps on the state line, with detainees living in tents he had requested as a loan from the War Department. Only after he was assured that travelers and their belongings were not infected with plague would they be allowed entry into neighboring states.

That afternoon, a Mrs. Peace, an elderly white woman from San Francisco on her way to Philadelphia, became one of the first train passengers removed, after an inspector at Truckee noticed her coughing and found that she did not have a signed health certificate. While the woman sat in detention, Kinyoun justified the policy by telling reporters that "The city and country have no protection against the plague which we know has caused at least twelve deaths among Chinese residents."

Consumed with containing the disease, Kinyoun had given no thought to how his order would be received by politicians and the press in a state which already distrusted him. The unilateral move to essentially seal the state seemed to confirm the worst stereotypes of him as an out-of-touch, vengeful man who knew no limits to his authority. Governor Gage sent telegrams to every contact he had in Washington, demanding that the Marine Hospital Service rescind the order at once and the federal government pay for any economic damage the state suffered as a result of Kinyoun's actions. William M. Cutter, a state senator, sent a personal message to President McKinley that read in part, "The indignation of the people of California is beyond expression. They protest in the strongest terms against this unjust and most unwarranted order and ask you at once direct its immediate revocation." Republican members of the state's congressional delegation, then in Philadelphia for the party's national convention, walked out of the proceedings and traveled to Washington, where they insisted upon a White House conference with President McKinley to warn him that every minute he allowed Kinyoun's quarantine to stand would increase the likelihood that he would lose the state in the upcoming presidential election. "Kinyoun should be mobbed, for his conduct is outrageous," said Douglas S. Cone, a prominent farmer and member of the delegation, as he boarded a train to the nation's capital. "There is no plague in California and no power on Earth could keep us still under these circumstances."

The press, which had fallen into the habit of referring to Kinyoun as "Suspicious Kinyoun" at every reference, eviscerated him. Blockading the state "is not a power to be exercised by some little whippersnapper whom political pull have invested with official authority. The only question now is as to what the President will do with this creature, and how soon he will do it," the *Chronicle* wrote in an editorial. The paper followed the next day with an essay that began, "If Dr. Kinyoun were the ablest physician and the most skillful bacteriologist in the world, instead of a person of no particular professional capacity, he would still be totally unfit for any official position involving responsibility, by reason of his self-sufficiency, imperiousness, lack of common sense, and pig-headed obstinacy."

Kinyoun had no one to lean on as the city and state turned further against him. Frank L. Coombs, the U.S. District Attorney and a close confidant of Governor Gage, called him the morning he issued the quarantine with a warning. Kinyoun was clearly disobeying Judge Morrow's injunction blocking the Marine Hospital Service from interfering in the state, he said, and should revoke his order immediately if he wished to avoid jail. Kinyoun refused to do so unless ordered to by either Wyman or the Secretary of the Treasury, neither of whom had made contact since he informed them of his intentions.

Hours later, Wong Wai, one of the merchants whom Kinyoun had stopped at the Ferry Building that morning, filed a complaint in the U.S. District Court accusing Kinyoun of violating Judge Morrow's orders by specifically targeting Asians. Morrow demanded that Kinyoun appear before the court and answer to a charge of contempt. Expecting to be vindicated, Kinyoun wired Wyman to ask who the Service planned to tap to defend him—only to learn in a terse dispatch from Washington that it would be Coombs. The Surgeon General offered no words of support for Kinyoun as the world crashed down upon him, directing him only to "be guided by [Coombs's] advice in all quarantine procedures."

With no choice other than to rely upon a man he considered an enemy, Kinyoun appeared at Coombs's office later that day. Before Kinyoun could ask how he planned to conduct his defense, Coombs told him that he would be lucky to receive just a six-month jail sentence. When Kinyoun interjected that he believed that he was fulfilling the responsibilities of his position, Coombs shouted him down, repeating that there was no legal ground for him to stand on and that he should plead guilty. Kinyoun left the meeting convinced "all the more that the District Attorney was playing a game in which it was his deliberate intention to make me the scapegoat and shoulder all the responsibility of the affair upon me," he later wrote in a letter to a friend.

The next day, President McKinley met with members of California's congressional delegation along with John D. Spreckels, the owner of the *San Francisco Call*, a Republican power broker whose sprawling empire in San Diego made him one of the wealthiest men in the state. In a short conference in the Oval Office, the President apologized for Kinyoun's actions and promised that he would order the Marine Hospital Service to revoke them at once. Minutes later, Wyman sent a telegram to Kinyoun that said simply, "Withdraw all inspections until further orders."

With that, Kinyoun's last hope was gone. He was in all respects powerless, unable to take any measures to confront the disease he remained convinced would soon overtake the nation. The uniform he had worn for nearly all of his professional life felt like nothing more than a monument to his failures. At Angel Island, the few officers with whom he remained on friendly terms began to distance themselves from him, as if trying to avoid catching the illness of defeat.

His professional life in ruins, Kinyoun narrowed his objective to staying out of jail. He appeared in court before Judge Morrow and promised that he would in no way target the Chinese or interfere in the right of open travel. Morrow refused to drop the contempt charge and ordered Kinyoun back the following week for trial, a one-year sentence hanging over his head. With Coombs urging him to plead guilty, Kinyoun sent increasingly desperate telegrams to Wyman, begging for new representation. "Still believe district attorney wholly inimical to interests of Surgeon-General, Marine-Hospital Service and Surgeon Kinyoun because refusal to have my actions fully investigated by court in contempt proceedings. Must renew request yesterday [for] additional counsel, and most respectfully insist direct orders," he wrote. After Wyman responded with a curt note that said he did not understand the reason why Coombs was insufficient, Kinyoun wrote another telegram begging for help. "I am convinced the decision of the court will be adverse. I therefore most respectfully demand full and adequate protection be accorded me by my Department. . . . If this is done I have no fear of the result. Being now placed in a position wherein I am deprived from protection of counsel I am forced to make this request."

Wyman was unswayed, maintaining an icy remove that pushed Kinyoun further into despair. His reputation was shattered, his sense of purpose lost. Reading a wire from Wyman a few days later informing him that culture samples that he had taken from suspected plague patients and sent to Washington for inspection in the Service's laboratory had been found to be genuine cases of plague was no balm for his bruised pride. The confirmation that he had been right all along was just one more insult, a little extra salt that made his wound sting all the more.

He had only to look at his children to see the toll that the year in California had taken on them. There was no school on Angel Island for them to attend, giving them no friends or distractions to serve as buffers from the stress that consumed his life. His oldest son, Conrad, could focus on little except the poor treatment of his father, making the boy seem prematurely aged. "He not only has old ways but old thoughts, and looks old in the bargain. Life to him is a very serious problem, and I often feel sorry for him," Kinyoun confessed in a letter back home. One night at the dinner table, Conrad remarked out of the blue that "Judge Morrow don't seem to know who my papa is; Judge Morrow thinks he's the biggest man in the world, but right there he's mistaken, he don't know my papa like I do," leaving Kinyoun heartbroken that the twelve-year-old felt he had to defend him.

By chance Kinyoun spotted Morrow on a ferry to Tiburon, a village on the northern edge of the bay, a few days before his trial was set to begin. He approached the judge and the two sat down near the stern as the boat cast off from the dock. Over the next forty minutes, Kinyoun detailed his experience of hunting plague in Chinatown, growing more animated as the ship picked up speed and fought against the wind of the open bay. "I am more and more convinced that the disease is behaving just exactly as it has in all other places after its introduction," Kinyoun told him. Morrow listened intently, for the first time hearing evidence of the plague's existence in the city that had been successfully excluded by attorneys for the Chinese Six Companies during previous trials. As the ferryboat approached shore, Morrow told Kinyoun that in the future he should meet with him personally on any legal questions before issuing orders, and promised to give him as much leeway to combat the disease as the law allowed.

In court days later, Kinyoun formally asked for clemency and pledged that he would not implement any further quarantine measures without the consent of Governor Gage. Morrow, in turn, ruled that there was insufficient evidence to hold Kinyoun in contempt of court for intentionally discriminating against the Chinese. Kinyoun

exited the courtroom a free but chastened man, unsure of his purpose in a city and state that was open in its hatred of him. Even if
he remained in his job, his ability to do anything to combat plague
was severely constrained, leaving him feeling as if he was nothing
more than an ornament. The disease was still there, lurking, and all
Kinyoun could now do was watch.

With Kinyoun sidelined, San Francisco was once again free to
believe that plague did not exist within its limits. The number of
suspected cases reported to the city Board of Health plummeted, as
if all the heat had gone out from a fire. No public updates on the
disease were issued by city medical officials, further smothering the
truth. Under pressure from the White House, the Marine Hospital
Service stopped publishing Kinyoun's detailed descriptions of plague
victims and his estimates of how many additional patients likely had
contracted the disease in *Public Health Reports*, its weekly dispatches
that were read by every government health officer in the country.

Letters from concerned doctors across the country began arriving
at Angel Island, asking Kinyoun for any new information. He felt
a duty to answer every one, even as it drained what little energy he
had left. Without him there to act as a counterbalance, physicians
affiliated with the Chinese Six Companies—men he called "nothing
more or less than vampires"—were free to attribute an increasing
number of deaths to kidney disease, a practice Kinyoun believed was
part of a conspiracy to hide plague victims. "I am almost at the point
sometimes of stating that plague will exist in Chinatown until the
district, now occupied by the Chinese, has been depopulated and
destroyed," Kinyoun wrote in a bitter letter that summer.

On August 11, William Murphy, a thirty-four-year-old team-
ster, died at City and County Hospital. The man had lived at 427
Dupont Street, just blocks outside Chinatown. He had been admitted to the hospital four days earlier complaining of a high fever and
mysterious headache that would not go away. Doctors discovered

a dark bubo on his right groin, an unmistakable sign of plague. From discussions with his relatives, they learned that Murphy had become addicted to morphine and was known to frequent Chinatown's opium dens. The doctors on call when Murphy died ordered an autopsy. With several professors from the city's medical schools looking on, the procedure revealed a body ravaged by a disease that authorities refused to admit was present in the city. Murphy's lymph nodes were hard and swollen, as if marbles lay under his skin. The tips of his fingers and toes were black—a sign of tissue decay that gave the medieval plague epidemics the name of the Black Death. Most frightening, the man's lungs were consumed by plague bacilli, indicating that the disease had progressed to the rare pneumonic stage, in which it could be spread by coughing alone.

Kinyoun felt no vindication as the disease claimed its first white victim. "This last case takes it out of the pale of Chinatown," he wrote in a letter to a friend on the East Coast. "The true nature of the issue was not known until the post-mortem examination revealed its true condition. I have just about completed the examination of specimens obtained from this last case and have no hesitancy in saying that it is the most beautiful case of plague infection (if such things can be called beautiful) that I have encountered in this epidemic."

Still the city denied the danger that it was in. Newspapers did not elaborate on the cause of Murphy's death and politicians ignored it. Neither the city or state Board of Health took further action to contain the disease despite undeniable evidence that it had breached the barriers of Chinatown. Soon more residents fell victim. Over the following four weeks, city Board of Health officials discovered six confirmed cases in Chinatown, including the body of Yung Wah Noui, a nine-year-old Chinese girl who had watched her mother, Moon Li Chee Yung, die from plague the day before. Yet nothing seemed enough to shake the city out of its complacency as its population continued to grow.

Soon hospitals were no longer safe. Anne Roede, a twenty-year-

old-white nurse, fell victim while working in the isolation ward of
Children's Hospital in San Francisco. An autopsy revealed a prominent bubo in her left armpit. As she lay dying, Roede refused to
answer a health officer's questions about her life before she contracted the disease, leaving them with no obvious connections to
Chinatown. Her death marked the twenty-first confirmed fatality
from plague in the eight months since Wong Chut King's body was
found in the Globe Hotel, though the true number was undoubtedly higher.

Kinyoun's warnings were slowly coming true, though the city
refused to listen. Instead of confronting the disease, it looked for ways
to further disguise the danger. As plague spread, Governor Gage
and his allies feared that Kinyoun would once again violate Morrow's orders despite the jail time that would be sure to follow. What
the governor needed was a way to remove Kinyoun from his post,
silencing him permanently. That October, he saw an opportunity.

The *Coptic*, a vessel in the Occidental and Oriental Steamship
Company line, sailed into San Francisco Bay from Hawaii and docked
at Angel Island for inspection. Quarantine officers approached it
with trepidation. Earlier that summer, the same ship had left San
Francisco bound for Honolulu. There it picked up passengers,
including a twenty-seven-year-old farmer by the name of Ah Sow,
and continued on its journey to Kobe, Japan. As it approached port,
passengers alerted the ship's doctor that Ah Sow had fallen into a
stupor. Officers found the man suffering from a fever above 105
degrees and discovered a black lump the size of an egg on his right
thigh. The man died shortly after he was carried ashore, becoming
the first known case of bubonic plague on a westbound ship that had
departed from the United States or its territories. In order to avert
a quarantine of its ports now that the plague had been eradicated
from Honolulu, health officials in Hawaii argued that rats that had
boarded the ship in San Francisco must have infected the man.

The ship itself was fumigated and doused with chemicals, and with a new crew continued on its return trip across the Pacific. Though its captain reported no illnesses aboard, quarantine officers took few chances as it neared Angel Island. Passengers were separated by gender and ordered to go into the ship's smoking rooms and strip for bodily inspection. First-class passengers found themselves standing naked next to men and women from third-class bunks. Marine Health Service officers went from person to person examining groins and armpits, searching for evidence of plague. Only when every person was cleared were the ship's passengers free to board ferries for San Francisco.

Complaints about the indelicate treatment were amplified in the press. Passengers vowed to never again sail into the port of San Francisco as long as Kinyoun was in charge of Angel Island, blaming him for the actions of his officers. The *Chronicle* ran a headline that asked "Has Kinyoun Gone Mad?" At the moment, he was nearly a thousand miles away in Vancouver, British Columbia, on an unrelated assignment. Governor Gage called the incident evidence that Kinyoun's "disregard for the welfare of the state" had filtered down to his staff. Unaware of the trouble brewing, Kinyoun returned to the city and resumed his post. A few days later, he ordered a Chinese ship carrying live animals into quarantine, citing their potential to carry the germs of plague. Such short-term detention was to be expected when hauling live cargo, and shipping companies often built in extra travel time in anticipation. This time, however, Kinyoun's enemies pounced. The president of the San Francisco Chamber of Commerce, Charles Nelson, publicly berated Kinyoun for his interference, labeling him "a menace to our trade and commerce." A bill was introduced in the state senate in Sacramento calling upon President McKinley to relieve Kinyoun from his position and prohibit him from setting foot in any city on the Pacific Coast. When criticized by a fellow state senator that the bill sentenced a federal health officer without trial, its author, William Cutter, declared on the floor of the senate that Kinyoun deserved to be hanged for his attempt to ban any outward travel from California. "Even now this man of black and malignant heart asserts that bubonic plague still exists in San Francisco. There is not a day in which Kinyoun may not impose another quarantine on the state," he said. After a few days of deliberation, the bill passed.

Gage, in his annual address to the state legislature in Sacramento, devoted a third of his nearly twenty-thousand-word speech to what he saw as Kinyoun's treachery. The number of tourists visiting San Francisco had plummeted in the days following Kinyoun's short-lived travel ban, he said, while the reputation of the state's produce had fallen so low that merchants in other states were now hanging banners stating "No California Fruits for Sale." All for a disease that had never been proven to exist in the state, Gage thundered. "Dr. Kinyoun, who has been so persistently obstinate in his reports of plague, never had any experience with the disease proper, his experience being derived wholly from books and laboratory work and not from practice among victims of the plague," he said, challenging not only Kinyoun personally but the ability of any bacteriologist to use microscopes and cultures to determine what the naked eye could not.

Like other so-called modern advances that had come out of New York or Europe, the science of bacteriology was suspect in his eyes, another step forward into a future in which an individual's own good sense was no longer considered enough. Regardless of whether an individual doctor could be trusted with these new and unproven tools, importing the germs responsible for deadly diseases, even for study, was fraught with the chance that they could be used for evil, Gage continued. "Who can tell what unscrupulous or negligent men, scientific or otherwise, might not do while possessing plague bacilli and knowing how to use the same?" he said, the implication that Kinyoun was among the corps of dangerous men all but shouted. Gage proposed a penalty of life imprisonment for any person who brought plague bacilli into the state or took tissue samples from a suspected plague victim with the intent to make a culture from it without the permission of the Governor. If it passed, the bill would silence not only Kinyoun but any future bacteriologist who tried to confirm the existence of plague in the state without being preselected by Gage or his successors.

Gage's campaign against the new era of science was not over. He announced that he would back legislation that would make it a felony to publish anything that suggested that bubonic plague was present in the state. "The circulation of such untrustworthy publications disseminated the plague scare broadcast, and wrought much of the injury which the people of the State have sustained. No state should permit such an outrage to be committed against its citizens by any man, set of men, or corporation," he said.

Under his proposals, the whole of public health—from its methods of study to its procedures of examination to its responsibility to report its findings—would be moved out of the realm of fact and into politics, a practice that the *Occidental Medical Times*, a medical journal in the state, found appalling. "The absurdity and falsity of these statements is most apparent, and the charge is a serious one," it wrote in an editorial. "If allowed to stand unchallenged, it will destroy all influence and power of medical opinion in California, and render similar evidence of the existence of disease null and void."

Kinyoun, who stubbornly refused to leave San Francisco until he was vindicated, could no longer contain himself under the assault. He wrote to Wyman, demanding that the Marine Hospital Service conduct an independent investigation into the existence of plague in San Francisco in order to clear his name and his reputation. "Governor has by implication charged me [with] being accessory to inoculating dead bodies with imported plague germs in order to foist upon community plague scare," Kinyoun wrote in a telegram. "Great stress now being laid [on] press dispatch from Washington stating that Surgeon-General has no longer any confidence in reports sent by me regarding plague here, as no further mention is made in Public Heath Reports, I [am] being disgraced and discredited." Wyman responded with a short telegram assuring Kinyoun that the Service had not lost its faith in him despite the governor's speech, which persuaded Kinyoun, for one of the few times in his life, to refrain from making a public show of his anger. "Kinyoun exercises more self-restraint than I thought possible," a fellow Marine Hospital surgeon in San Francisco privately wrote to Wyman.

Yet Wyman did not know that Kinyoun had already turned his fire against the man he blamed for upending his life's path. He sent a private letter to Francis Cockerel, the sitting U.S. senator from his home state of Missouri, requesting his assistance. The presence of plague "has been proven by every test that science demands, and has been confirmed by some of the best bacteriologists in the United States," he wrote. Now, he said, it was time for Wyman to fully support him and repay his years of service. "My exoneration rests upon Dr. Wyman openly avowing his responsibility for my official actions. This he should, and will do, if he possesses the courage of a man, and wishes to do what is honorable . . . All these years I have stood loyally by the side of Dr. Wyman, fought hard his battles, shielded him in his mistakes, and propped up many of his weak-kneed policies, and on more than one occasion used my best efforts, and not without success, in keeping his political head from rolling into the basket," he wrote.

All the while, the number of deaths continued to rise. Three confirmed cases of the disease were discovered over the first two weeks of 1901, bringing the unofficial death total to twenty-five. Among them were Angelo Colombo, an immigrant from Switzerland who lived at 5 Lafayette Place, a building a half mile south of City Hall that was more than a forty-minute walk from Chinatown. A police officer on patrol had discovered the man lying unconscious with a high fever, and a subsequent autopsy revealed black marks on his feet and hands and plague bacilli in his bloodstream. With Kinyoun's urging, Wyman announced that he would send a team of three independent doctors with no federal affiliation to San Francisco to settle the question of whether plague existed in the city. Their findings were expected to be published in medical journals nationally, ending months of rumors.

Kinyoun waited for the public exoneration that he felt was his due, knowing that his professional survival was at stake. He was at war with everyone in California, he wrote in a letter to an East Coast friend, and could only console himself with thinking that his enemies would receive their punishments in the end. "I believe that the old Jewish law is right," he wrote. "We know surely, that if we transgress the law of nature we pay the penalty, and if you do someone wrong, the same will be meted out to you in the end. While I do not wish to visit retribution upon those who have been so short-sighted as to cause innocent people to suffer, I am sure that such will occur sooner or later."

CHAPTER 8

AN INFAMOUS COMPACT

The room was filled with empty seats. On January 26, 1901, three graying scientists stared out into an elegant ballroom at the Occidental Hotel in San Francisco. The men had traveled across the continent, having been appointed by officials in Washington to serve on a commission "for the purpose of ascertaining the existence or non-existence of bubonic plague in the city of San Francisco." As a show of the transparency of their inquiry, they had pledged to hold open meetings at the hotel every morning at eleven o'clock, where anyone with information to share or an interest in the proceedings could take a seat. As their first meeting began, they gazed out upon only a handful of spectators.

Sitting at a long table in the front of the room were Simon Flexner, a professor of pathology at the University of Pennsylvania, Frederick Novy, an assistant professor of bacteriology at the University of Michigan, and Lewellys Barker, a professor of anatomy at the University of Chicago. All had had firsthand experience of the disease in India. Flexner and Barker, in addition, had independently sailed to the Philippines and Hong Kong and evaluated the methods doctors used in treating plague victims there. Though he did not have a personal relationship with any of the men, Kinyoun was well aware of their professional reputations and considered them his peers. Had he chosen a life of academic study over the treatment of patients in the Marine Hospital Service, he could have very well been sitting in their spots, his rough edges perhaps sanded away by the assurance that he was respected.

As the lone bacteriologist in the group, it was Novy who instead represented the coming age of laboratory science. Kinyoun hoped that the man's high reputation and professional air would make the commission's findings unassailable, even as Novy followed the same techniques and procedures that he had followed in his laboratory on Angel Island. Privately, Novy had his doubts. "The Governor of California denies the existence of the disease in San Francisco," he wrote in a letter to his wife, Grace, shortly after arriving in the city. "The press and people are unanimously against the idea that plague exists here . . . The newspapers and governor feel that they must not be guided by bacteriological evidence. They will in the end lambaste us just as they have done to Kinyoun should we find plague."

The presence of more outsiders was the last thing Governor Gage wanted. Before the commission members arrived, the *Occidental Medical Times*, the most powerful medical journal on the West Coast, announced that doctors outside San Francisco considered their work above reproach and were prepared to accept their findings without question. "They are men whose knowledge and integrity are beyond impeachment by the chief executive or the newspapers of this state, and we trust that their verdict will settle for all times the most disgraceful, most pitiable, and the most humiliating chapter in the medico-political history of California," it noted in an editorial. The commission members, meanwhile, were determined not to make the same mistakes as Kinyoun and focused on presenting a humble, open face to the city. "We are now at work, seeking only the truth," Barker said during his first meeting with the press.

Governor Gage had tried to stifle the inquiry before it began. After officials in Washington named the commission officers, he sent a wire to President McKinley complaining that he had not been allowed a hand in selecting its members. "I hope that in this matter of vital interest to the people of California there is no intentional discourtesy," he wrote. Unable to pack it with doctors he considered allies, the governor announced that he would not accept the commission's findings unless they could produce living patients with the disease, a feat that had long eluded Kinyoun. When the commission members arrived in San Francisco and began searching for laboratory space, Governor Gage ordered the president of the University of California to deny them use of facilities on campus and refused to meet with them in person, believing that by denying them recognition he could undercut their authority. The doctors were forced to turn an empty office in City Hall into a makeshift laboratory, purchasing microscopes and other vital equipment on the fly. Though Kinyoun offered supplies and assistance, the commission officers rejected them, not wanting the appearance of association that could later be used to cast doubt on their work. The small room in City Hall was soon packed with instruments, leaving no suitable space for autopsies. In the coming weeks, the men had to conduct the procedures in funeral homes and in the rooms where bodies were found.

Their laboratory complete, the doctors took their first tour of Chinatown, accompanied by police officers. The district was "shockingly unsanitary," they would later write. Its "rooms are small; they are often entirely devoid of light or means of ventilation . . . many of them are filthy; some of them, especially those situated in basements, are damp and emit a foul stench." Prostitution was rife, allowing venereal disease to spread without constraint. Yet even so, they noted with grim irony, the rooms in which the prostitutes lived were "on the whole, more wholesome in some regards [such as] air space, light, ventilation and cleanliness than those of the other inhabitants of the district."

On their tenth day in San Francisco, they found their first plague victim. The body of Chu Ah Chon, a forty-four-year-old actor, was discovered in a room above a theater at 814 Washington Street and carted to a nearby undertaker's shop. The commission members examined the corpse in a dimly lit back room. Large bluish spots, a sign of internal bleeding that was often present on plague victims in India, dotted the man's legs, while the glands in the neck, groin and armpits bulged. Typically, such clear evidence of plague would have pressed the doctors into conducting an immediate autopsy. Yet owing to the protests of their Chinese interpreter, who voiced his revulsion at any form of bodily mutilation, they agreed to make only the minimal incisions required to take tissue samples. They rushed the material back to their City Hall laboratory, where Novy, like Kinyoun before him, inoculated a guinea pig with cultures he isolated from the man's body. The animal soon developed symptoms of plague and died a few days later, confirming that Chu was the twenty-sixth known victim of the epidemic. "Plague was present beyond possible doubt," Novy wrote in his notebook.

Perhaps recognizing that the men he was now working with were more willing to respect Chinese customs than Kinyoun, who would concede nothing in his search for medical evidence, their interpreter soon informed them of several people suffering from apparent plague symptoms whose identities were known to the Chinese Six Companies but who had remained hidden from Western health officials. The commission members examined more than a dozen patients, marking the first time that living carriers of the disease were officially recorded.

Tom Shon, a fifty-one-year-old male actor and the roommate of Chu Ah Chon, seemed lost in a stupor of delirium when the commission doctors arrived at his apartment. Surprised that the man was still alive, Barker examined him. His skin was hot and dry to the touch and he winced when doctors put pressure on the enlarged glands in his groin. Though there were no buboes present, Barker told the man's friends that a dose of the Haffkine serum was the only hope for his survival, though he cautioned that it might be too late. Shon's friends refused the offer and he died the following morning. Tissues taken during a partial autopsy revealed plague.

Days later, the doctors descended into a cramped and filthy hovel at 921 Dupont Street. There they found Ng Ah Bock, a forty-five-year-old Chinese man who had been ill for two weeks with a high fever. Though friends present said that his mind no longer seemed anchored in reality, the man felt well enough to attempt a conversation as Barker began examining him and soon discovered a dark bubo bulging from his neck. The next day, Ng's body was found outside a coffin shop on Sacramento Street, apparently dumped there by the men Baker had conversed with in the tiny shared apartment. An autopsy confirmed that he had died of bubonic plague.

Not all cases were as obvious. Fong Ah Fong, a twelve-year-old girl living at 747 Sacramento Street, showed no outward signs of plague when the doctors first examined her. The girl had been ill with a low fever for two weeks, her mother said, yet her temperature had not spiked and there was no evidence of inflammation in her glands. Suspecting that it was not plague and more likely a mild case of typhoid, the doctors asked her mother to contact them if the girl got worse. She died a few days later. Confused by the sudden decline, the commission members returned to the apartment to examine the body. Finding no buboes, they pressed her mother to allow them to conduct an autopsy, explaining that it was the only way they could determine if the girl had contracted the disease and where the infection had been hiding in her body.

The room suddenly filled with angry men and women, all violently objecting. Facing what he later called "an appalling outbreak of grief," Barker promised to make only one small incision in the groin of the dead girl in order to capture a tissue sample, which confirmed that she had indeed died from plague. "In the face of the strong protest made by the friends, it seemed wise not to antagonize the Chinese too much, and so interfere with the progress of the whole investigation," Barker later wrote in the commission's official report, apologizing for what he called the limited anatomical evidence collected from victims.

Fong's death marked the sixth case of plague the commission

had identified in Chinatown within a single week and brought the official number of dead to twenty-six in ten months. Only two of the victims discovered by the commission developed buboes on their bodies, requiring Novy's laboratory work for a true determination of the cause of death. "It is difficult to make a diagnosis of plague without bacteriological examination," he later wrote. "In the absence of primary buboes, the unskilled observer will miss practically every case, and even the practitioner who has had much experience with plague may be deceived."

While unanimous in their belief that plague was indeed endemic in Chinatown, the doctors nevertheless remained puzzled. In every other outbreak of the disease, plague had spread "like a great tidal wave with unusual force," Novy wrote. Yet in San Francisco it remained constrained by some invisible hand, even if the true death toll was likely far higher than the official record. An unknown factor was saving the city from devastation, but none of the doctors could even guess at what it was. Their only hope was that the disease would continue its strange pattern until a sanitation campaign could fully eradicate it, sparing San Francisco from the devastation they had seen in India.

The commission members met privately with Governor Gage at the Palace Hotel. Plague was indeed spreading within the city, they told him, and they had witnessed it in victims before their deaths, a phenomenon that Gage considered impossible. The governor grew irate, accusing the men of infecting victims with plague themselves through their careless handling of germs. He demanded to know whether they had been influenced by Kinyoun, and raged even more when told that Kinyoun was not involved. Shortly before they left the meeting, the doctors told the governor that they were close to finishing a full report that would confirm the presence of the disease in San Francisco which they would send to Washington in the coming days.

Governor Gage immediately wired a letter of protest to the Treasury Department, which at the time oversaw all matters of public health, railing against the publication of an investigation he called "unjust" and "unfair." Should the document make its way around Washington and into the hands of a reporter, Gage knew that the state's economy—still dependent on its reputation as a mythical land apart from the ordinary concerns of the nation—would collapse. "Whatever differences of opinion may at this time exist as to the existence or non-existence of plague, no one can honestly be of the opinion that the disease is epidemic in San Francisco, nor can anybody seriously contend that ample protective and preventative measures cannot be taken in the premises without even spreading great or any alarm among the people and without disturbing our commercial affairs," Gage wrote. He followed it up with a second telegram, in which he demanded a private meeting between the congressional representatives of the state and Surgeon General Wyman before the report was publicly released.

Gage did not know it, but he was not alone in his attempt to keep the truth from spreading. In Washington, Wyman was also intent on suppressing the news circulating among medical researchers that the disease had been confirmed in California. Worrying that a wire service reporter would pick up on the rumors and write an article that would be reprinted across the country, Wyman refused to talk about the commission's findings with his subordinates, even though he trusted that plague was indeed in the city as they had described. He instead harbored a hope that with delay and denial he could "bring the Governor around to work with us," he wrote in a private letter to a colleague, making the task of eradicating the disease easier. His greatest fear was that a copy of the full report would be published, further inflaming a man intent on making it impossible to conduct modern medicine in his state.

In San Francisco, Gage arranged a confidential meeting of the city's power brokers. The editors of San Francisco's largest papers, the president of the Pacific Mail Steamship Company, and attorneys for the Southern Pacific Railway—a group that collectively controlled the news that San Franciscans read, the goods that appeared on their docks and the trains that connected them with the nation—listened as Gage described the harm that publication of the commission's report would pose to their futures. He had each man present promise to refrain from republishing or acknowledging any reports issued by the plague commission, even after they were released by the federal government.

Assured of a news blackout, Gage then assembled a delegation that immediately headed to Washington to press for the permanent suppression of the commission's report and any federal mention of the plague in California. The group included the editors of the *San Francisco Chronicle*, the *San Francisco Bulletin* and the *San Francisco Examiner*, the chief counsel for the Southern Pacific Railway and the president of Union Iron Works, who happened to be a close friend of President McKinley. Unlike the secret pact among the newspapers to hide the news of plague, the men Gage picked boasted that they intended to rid the city of the federal health officers who had caused problems for too long. As he boarded the train for Washington, John P. Young, the editor of the *Chronicle*, announced that he would return with "Kinyoun's scalp dangling from his belt."

Surgeon General Wyman met with the California delegation and presented them with copies of the commission's final report, which had yet to be published. It concluded that plague was not only in San Francisco, but had likely been in the city for at least two years. The doctors could point to no reason why the city had thus far been spared the epidemics that had wasted Bombay and Hong Kong, yet they remained certain that it was only a matter of time. And San Francisco was not the only city at risk. The inability of health officers to forcefully confront the disease had most likely allowed it to expand to other large cities, including Sacramento and Los Angeles. If the disease was not confronted, the report declared, an epidemic could soon envelop the country.

The findings were plain, and sobering. Faced with hard evidence that the plague was not a hoax or the result of Kinyoun mishandling tissue, the California delegation abandoned its efforts to undermine the doctors who had served on the commission. While careful to maintain that they did not officially acknowledge the report's findings, the delegation offered a bargain: the city and state would pay for a full sanitation campaign in Chinatown which would identify and treat plague victims and eliminate any trace of the disease, in exchange for the promise that the commission's findings were never made public. After all, they argued, the only thing that could save lives now was the sort of sanitary response that Marine Health Service officials had long wanted but had never had the support of the city or state to conduct; why make the process more difficult by publishing a report that could lead to panic? Sensing that the deal offered a chance for his agency to save face in California, as well as quelling an open challenge to his agency's federal authority, Wyman agreed, assuring the delegation that the commission's report would not be published while he remained Surgeon General.

Left unsaid was that Kinyoun would never go along with such a plan. Before the meeting was over, Wyman told the men from California to consider Surgeon Joseph White, one of his senior agents, the officer now in charge of the Angel Island post. He then composed a telegram to Kinyoun informing him that he was being transferred to Detroit. There would be none of the public vindication that Kinyoun had desperately sought, but Wyman counseled him to put the duty of his office to save lives ahead of his pride. "The conferences have been harmonious, without personal or other accusations being made, and cooperation of all concerned is assured," he wrote. "Public exigency requires personal feelings and any desire on part of Bureau [the Marine Health Service] or any others for public verification of statements made or position taken must be subordinated to maintain the present attitude of non-publication, even though outsiders may have published some facts not obtained through Bureau. The Department and the Bureau and its officers will maintain this attitude until further orders."

Kinyoun considered it Wyman's final betrayal. This time, however, Wyman's duplicity had not only hurt him personally but harmed millions of unsuspecting men and women across the country who did not know that the Surgeon General was complicit in a plan to keep the truth from them. Kinyoun believed in a future where scientists like him had rendered the concept of infectious disease moot, sparing the lives of innocent people. Instead, he had to face a present in which politics mattered more than honesty, and ignorance proved more powerful than medicine. "All this goodwill wiped out at the insistence of a few politicians is not only humiliating to the officers of this service, but a calamity to the nation," he wrote to a friend.

Despite Wyman's best efforts, a copy of the commission's report was leaked from the Marine Hospital Service and reached the *Occidental Medical Times*, which published it in full. The *Sacramento Bee* then revealed the secret meeting in Washington that had kept the Marine Hospital Service from publishing the report, calling it an "infamous compact." Medical officials were shocked to read not only the details of how plague had established itself in a major city, but that San Francisco had thus far been successful in concealing it from its own citizens. With Wyman's blessing, the federal government had intentionally helped California deceive the country, allowing thousands of Americans to travel to the state unaware that they were putting their families in danger. Their trust in California broken, health authorities in other states began preparing quarantine measures that they hoped would prevent plague from spilling across their borders. "I have but little conference in the California authorities, and unless I have a positive assurance from you that this State will be carefully protected by you from the disease I shall immediately order the most stringent quarantine regulations," wrote Joseph

D. Sayers, the governor of Texas, in a personal telegram to Wyman. "Please answer, by wire, immediately, as I will take no risk."

Though his deception was now well known, Wyman refused to apologize. He had done what he considered necessary to coerce California into funding the costly cleanup campaign it needed, and that, and nothing else, was what would protect the country. "To secure this harmonious action and its continuance I have felt convinced of the necessity of not giving out for publication all the facts in the case," Wyman wrote in a letter to state health authorities across the nation. In a gesture of openness, he enclosed with it one of Kinyoun's reports on the spread of the epidemic in San Francisco that he had previously pulled from the weekly *Public Health Reports* bulletin. "By avoiding unnecessary publicity I feel that the actual necessary work has been and will be made possible and expedited," Wyman wrote, not allowing himself to feel shame.

As he counted down his final days in San Francisco, Kinyoun vowed to make the most of them. He accepted invitations to appear at medical societies throughout the state, where he spoke at length about his experience fighting to be heard in a city that did not wish to acknowledge reality. In front of packed halls of doctors and public health officers who had never seen plague, he discussed how the disease presents itself in the body as a victim edges closer to death. He confessed that he did not understand why the city's death toll was not much higher: in epidemics in Hong Kong and Sydney, it had taken no more than a year after the discovery of the first victims for the disease to show its full strength, and San Francisco was now already well past that point. The odd behavior of the disease, in which it appeared to select individual victims rather than flooding through a neighborhood, could change at any moment, he cautioned, and the city was still not prepared.

He grew the most animated when he returned to the harder truths he had learned. When he first arrived in California, he had expected that a city would always put its safety above its ambition, he said. Only now did he realize how naive that was. Any doctor who followed through on his public responsibility to report plague cases "must be prepared to be made a target by a subsidized press, to submit to all the lowest forms of persecution, simply because he has had no more sense than to do his duty and tell the truth," Kinyoun told an audience of doctors in Sacramento.

He then quoted none other than Wyman, from an address the Surgeon General had made the year before regarding cities that attempted to suppress reports of cholera. "It is inconsistent with every known law of God, of every principle of sound policy, and of well doing among men that an individual or a city or state can successfully protect itself behind the flimsy barrier of a lie, particularly in dealing with the phenomena of nature," Wyman had said. "If a case of cholera occurs in a city, and be hidden under the disguise of a simple intentional derangement, to avoid public clamor and injuries to the commerce and avenues of the state, the last hope of destroying the contagion is wiped away, and thousands of lives and the general ruin of industry must pay the penalty of a sordid, short-sighted, wretched policy." Kinyoun left it up to his audience to determine whether a lie to cover up the plague was somehow better than a lie to mask cholera.

There was no reason to believe that the state would follow through on its compromise with Wyman, Kinyoun warned. The plague commission had found six confirmed cases in less than a week during its short investigation, but there had been no new victims identified since the deal was struck in Washington and the Gage administration had already started to suggest that it might not fund the cleanup effort as promised. Plague was in San Francisco, and, like all truths, would spread whether California's doctors wanted to admit it or not. At the end of his speech, Kinyoun relayed a remark once made on the floor of the state senate by Senator Cutter, the man who had stated that Kinyoun should be hung for his attempt at quarantining the state. Only with Kinyoun's removal, Senator

Cutter said, could the people of San Francisco "sleep undisrupted, and by day follow their avocations without fear." Now that the state appeared to get what Cutter had wished for, California was free "to enjoy bubonic plague to its full fruition," Kinyoun said.

There was no disguising his bitterness. As he packed his belongings at Angel Island and prepared his family to move again, Kinyoun could only look back over the last year and a half with anger. He had once been a rising star who made his name by saving the lives of others; now he found himself once more headed to an inglorious posting, where none of his brilliance in the laboratory would matter, simply because he could not allow himself to play the game of politics if it meant watching people die and doing nothing. Even after his demotion, Kinyoun had continued to send reports to Washington estimating the spread of the disease. Wyman replied just once, telling him that all future communications should be sent via Joseph White.

Kinyoun considered resigning his post rather than appear comfortable with Wyman's deceptions, but he was swayed by the pleas of fellow Marine Hospital officers. "Don't do it, old man," wrote Henry Rose Carter, who had played a key part in establishing that mosquitoes spread yellow fever and who remained one of Kinyoun's closest friends. "You are one of the men who helped make this service . . . Believe me . . . Your life and good works will never be lost."

With his future in the Marine Hospital Service ruined, Kinyoun's sole consolation was the response of other medical professionals to his courage. "It is the well-studied plan of Dr. Wyman and in fact others to simply relegate me to oblivion, and because of the prominence which my laboratory work had been assuming in the past five or six years," Kinyoun wrote to a friend. "It is most natural for a weak man, such as Dr. Wyman appears to be, to resent any such prominence of his subordinates, and therefore desires to regulate us to places where we cannot be so prominently before the public. There is one thing, however, that Dr. Wyman nor anyone else in the Marine Hospital Service can take from me, and that is my professional standing and character. The medical journals all over the United States have really been unstinted in their praise of the attitude which I assumed regarding the [plague], and my actions in carrying out the laws and regulations, and I have the unqualified confidence, you may say, of the whole profession in the United States. That is to me of more value than any word of praise which could emanate from Dr Wyman, or anyone connected with the Marine Hospital Service."

San Francisco had one final humiliation waiting before it would let Kinyoun leave. On the day that he was scheduled to board a train eastward with his family, he was arrested while riding an early morning ferry to Tiburon. A deaf and mute man had come forward with a story that Kinyoun had fired several rounds from a rifle at his boat as it passed by Angel Island, each one barely missing his head and tearing holes in his sail. Police officers hustled Kinyoun before a judge that same morning to answer to a charge of attempted murder. Angry and stunned, Kinyoun testified that he had not fired the shots and instead had saved the man's life. Marine Hospital Service officers at Angel Island had noticed the boat and wrongly assumed that it carried an escapee from the nearby island prison of Alcatraz. Kinyoun, hearing the commotion, had raced out from his laboratory and ordered his men to stop shooting. The judge dismissed the charge, though the damage had been done.

Kinyoun had come to San Francisco expecting that he would continue to push science forward and help change the world; now he slunk away in defeat, with newspapers gleefully reporting on his arrest as if intent on seizing their one last chance to defame him. As he boarded a train that would take him away from a city he loathed, Kinyoun remained haunted by his failures. Plague was still there, and it was spreading. He prayed that whoever replaced him would find a way to accomplish what he could not.

CHAPTER 9

AN IMPOSSIBLE TASK

The breakdown started as soon as Kinyoun boarded the train heading east.

Joseph White, the man who replaced him, found his calls unreturned by city and state officials responsible for funding the cleanup the California delegation had agreed to in Washington. State health officials who had been placed under White's command began finding novel excuses to disobey orders, going so far as to claim that removing furniture from a building suspected of housing a plague victim was against city regulations. The Chinese Six Companies, meanwhile, dodged all efforts to bring in independent physicians to examine residents of Chinatown, though it had promised the Marine Hospital Service its full cooperation if Kinyoun was removed from his post. Every morning, White requested that the organization identify all sick residents of Chinatown for inspection by a doctor employed by his agency. The district's population of 15,000 would result in a sick rate of about 150 patients per day under ordinary circumstances, White estimated. Instead, the Six Companies pointed him to only two or three residents with minor illnesses, a gesture that White took as a greater insult than an outright denial of his request.

Though he had just taken command on Angel Island, White was rapidly losing hope. It was now clear to him that Kinyoun, while a constant source of irritation to the Surgeon General, and hated by everyone in power in San Francisco, had been the only person standing in the way of chaos. Wyman, sensing that the situation was rapidly deteriorating, assured White in a telegram that he would soon have reinforcements. He was assembling a team of the best officers in the Service, he promised, and they would arrive by the end of the month. Yet White believed that even with an infinite number of doctors at his disposal, the problem would not change. The gulf between the Chinese and white health officers was too large, with too much distrust on both sides, to ever be breached.

"I yesterday inspected rooms in the cellars of some of the worst districts, which I do not believe to have been entered before by any white man in many months, and some of these rooms, partially underground and separated from either street or alley by flanking rooms on either side, are absolutely devoid of light and ventilation, are filthy beyond anything that may be imagined by the Caucasian mind, and filled with a stifling odor suggesting months of opium smoking, with occasional urination upon the floors. I can best describe it by saying that it is the accentuated odor of a rat den," White wrote in a long letter to Wyman admitting he was overwhelmed by the amount of work that needed to be done. "This letter being only one for the information of the Bureau, I shall speak quite plainly about this matter, both as to inspection and disinfection, and say that from present appearances the thorough cleansing of Chinatown appears to be a lost physical impossibility, and that I am certain of the absolute dishonesty of the Chinese in the promises that they have made, and well satisfied that they will fulfill nothing that they can possibly avoid. I shall in this instance, as I have ever done, perform the duties assigned to me to the best of my ability, but feel that it is only justice not only to myself but to the Service to say that I do not feel hopeful regarding the results."

Wyman alerted White in the following days that he would soon have a deputy by the name of Rupert Blue, a thirty-two-year-old physician in the Marine Hospital Service who was then en route from Milwaukee. White did not know it, but Blue was neither Wyman's first or second choice to fill the role. Wyman had selected him only after other candidates had threatened to leave the Service rather than take on the impossible task. For Blue, the move would amount to something of a return voyage: he had worked in San Francisco briefly as a quarantine officer five years earlier, and had more familiarity with the city and its intricacies than most men in the Service. Despite that experience, Blue carried a reputation for laziness that soon reached White and soured him on a man he had never personally met.

Already feeling like he was leading a losing war, White wrote a blunt letter to Wyman requesting that Blue be replaced before he set foot in San Francisco. "The difficulties here are so great that never before in our history has there been a greater need for tactful and forceful officers and mediocrity is I think clean out of place," he wrote. "I learn that Blue has [no tact] and is inert beside. I don't know Blue and have not a reason under Heaven to dislike him, so there is nothing personal in this matter at all, but I am fully persuaded that he cannot take the lead in this matter now or in the future."

For all of his life, Rupert Blue had shouldered the weight of not meeting other people's expectations. The sixth of eight siblings, Blue was born on May 30, 1868, into a prominent Southern family still adrift three years after the end of the Civil War. His father, John Gilchrist Blue, had been a member of the North Carolina delegation that voted to secede from the Union, and then served as a colonel in the Confederate Army, fighting alongside Robert E. Lee in the Army of Northern Virginia until the surrender at Appomattox. When Rupert was three the family moved to Marion, South Carolina, in order to be closer to the home of Rupert's mother, Annie Maria Evans, whose family included past governors of the state. Thanks to their influence, the Blues were given a second start. John Gilchrist Blue settled his family into a 300-acre plantation he named Bluefields and opened a law practice. Before long he was elected to the South Carolina state legislature, which made him one of the most recognizable people in Marion.

Rupert grew up in a town small enough that everyone knew who his parents were, and in a family prominent enough that any misstep would be recounted in each one of the stately Greek Revival mansions that lined Marion's streets. A natural introvert with a slight stammer, he retreated from the watchful eyes of his neighbors and into the open expanses of the plantation, where along with his siblings he would sneak into the fields early in the morning and burst open melons with his fists before devouring them bare-handed. Though physically strong, growing to stand above six feet tall with a wide boxer's build that he would put to use in the ring later in life, Rupert could more often than not be found holed up alone with a book. The boy feasted on history, devouring any account of ancient Rome he could get his hands on, and soon developed a lifelong fascination with the military campaigns of Napoleon. Those reading sessions were as close as he would come to military service, however, and he chose to stand in the shadows as his older brother, Victor, took up a family tradition that included a grandfather who had served as a colonel in the War of 1812 and great-grandfathers who fought on opposing sides in the Revolutionary War.

It was soon clear that Victor was everything that Rupert was not. Though only two years apart, the boys seemed cut from different stone. Where Victor was outgoing, Rupert retreated; where Rupert was a great listener, Victor was bombastic, expecting that his natural charm would smooth over any wrinkles that life threw at him. Victor soon became "the family paragon, and entirely worthy of the great love his parents, brothers and sisters bore him," his sister Kate Lilly once wrote. "Rupert is very different. He just cannot stand on the street corner and give the glad hand to somebody he might have gone to school with."

Victor's decision to enter the military only brought him closer to his father, cementing his status as the favorite son. Rupert, indifferent to the pageantry of rank in the service, searched for another way to make a mark. He found it in the rapidly professionalizing world of medicine. The nation was growing and industrializing, and a new class of doctor was needed to care for it.

Smart young men were filling the halls of the hundreds of medical schools sprouting up across the country, drawn as much by the prospect of opening a lucrative private practice as by the promise of healing the sick. While the students received some exposure to the new sciences of bacteriology and immunology, most were content to become what was then known as a commercial physician, their degree essentially functioning as a pass that allowed them to set up a small general practice and be their own boss.

The boomtown nature of the field naturally brought uneven results. "These enterprises—for the most part, they can be called schools or institutions only by courtesy—were frequently set up regardless of opportunity or need, in small towns as readily as in large, and at times, almost in the heart of the wilderness," noted the *Atlantic* in a 1910 article about the transformation of medical education then happening in America. "Nothing was really essential but professors . . . little or no investment was therefore involved. A hall could be cheaply rented, and rude benches were inexpensive. Janitor service was unknown and is even now relatively rare. Occasional dissections in time supplied a skeleton—in whole or in part—and a box of odd bones. Other equipment there was practically none."

Rupert enrolled in a small medical school in Latta, South Carolina, studying what was then known as practical pharmacy. Despite a distance of just eleven miles from Marion—a length he could walk in a day if it came to it—he was painfully homesick, spending solitary nights in his boardinghouse room dreaming of the comfortable confines of Bluefields. He attempted to show a brave face to his family, unwilling to fall short once again of the standard that Victor had set. "Thanks to a nature that is cosmopolitan, I am content to live anywhere," he wrote in a letter, full of the bluster of a young man away from home for the first time.

That Christmas, his father suffered a heart attack, brought on by years of heavy tobacco use and the lingering damage from a childhood bout of rheumatic fever. Rupert rushed home to be at his side, and remained there until he died on January 6, 1889. His death changed something in Rupert, then just twenty-one years old. With his mother and two older unmarried sisters left with few resources and little income, he realized that there was no longer any place for boyhood. He vowed to provide for them as well as possible, in ways that Victor, whose military service flung him around the world, could not.

Rupert entered the University of Virginia at Charlottesville, determined to become a higher caliber of doctor, capable of commanding both money and respect. He willed himself to compete, wringing out the last of his retiring nature and replacing it with a sense of purpose that had long been lacking. He masked his newfound determination under the façade of a polite Southern gentleman, though his letters home left little doubt as to his new life's direction. "I will not assimilate the vices of others," he wrote to his sister Kate. "If I am spared to good health I can accomplish something for I have the will & the ambition."

Money remained so tight that in his letters home he crammed as many words onto a single sheet of paper as he could, not only filling the margins but sometimes flipping it sideways and continuing to write lengthwise until no blank spot was left. His lack of funds made courting a woman an impossibility, an embarrassment that he tried to hide from wealthier classmates. When fellow students assumed that a photo of his sister Kate hanging in his room was his girlfriend, Rupert readily went along with the ruse until "sophisticated-eyed Joe Guthrie detected the resemblance and gave the deception away," he wrote in a letter home. After two years, he moved farther north to Baltimore to enroll in the University of Maryland School of Medicine, the first public medical school in the country and one of the few that he could afford. Never a prodigy, Rupert got through the demanding program by grit alone, holing up in his room with wads of tobacco and devoting every moment to mastering the material. "I am working like a Trojan," he wrote in a letter home. "There is so much to learn."

In those lonely hours of study, Rupert slowly developed an ambition to become something greater than the common physician he had first imagined himself, focused more on the bottom line than on his patients' health. He had willed himself to get through medical school, and he did not want to feel that the effort was wasted. Victor was rising through the ranks of the military, and Rupert was determined not to be left behind again. The day after his graduation, he wrote a letter to Kate in which he spelled out the kind of doctor he hoped to be. "I begin my professional career today with perfect cognizance of the many responsibilities that rest upon my shoulders. When I listened to the valedictory address I mentally determined that I should ever be found on the side of the right—let the consequences be as they may."

He soon found a venue that supplied not only a way to provide for his family but the excitement that he had longed for as a boy. Upon graduation, he applied to the Marine Hospital Service, thrilled at the prospect of traveling to exotic locations and treating illnesses that he had only read about. "Infectious disease is one of the few genuine adventures left in the world," Hans Zinsser would later write in his influential *Rats, Lice and History*, a 1935 tract which described the state of the medical profession around the turn of the twentieth century. "The dragons are all dead, and the lance grows rusty in the chimney corner. Wars are exercises in ballistics, chemical ingenuity, administration, hard physical labour, and long-distance mass murder. . . . However secure and well-regulated civilized life may become, bacteria, protozoa, viruses, infected fleas, lice, ticks, mosquitoes, and bedbugs will always lurk in the shadows ready to pounce when neglect, poverty, famine, or war lets down the defenses."

Like Victor, Rupert was ready to travel the world and serve his country; unlike his brother, however, Rupert's purpose was to heal rather than to hurt. He soon learned that he was one of only four candidates to gain acceptance into the Service that year. He received an annual salary of $1,800—equivalent to roughly $50,000 in today's dollars—and began sending a hefty portion of every paycheck home to his mother and sisters. As he donned his dark gray Service uniform for the first time, he saw in his reflection the man he had always wanted to be.

One of his first postings sent him to investigate an outbreak of yellow fever in Galveston, Texas. The bustling coastal city sat on an island jutting into the Gulf of Mexico, separated from the mainland by a short bridge that connected the Texas of sagebrush and cowboys with the wider modern world. Over forty-five steamship lines provided direct connections to destinations ranging from New York to Europe, funneling people and goods into the busiest cotton port in the nation. Electric streetcars ran down its broad streets, passing ornate mansions. A jumble of nationalities and languages enlivened its stores and restaurants, creating a society so cosmopolitan that the *New York Herald* dubbed the city "New York on the Gulf."

It took weeks for Rupert to acclimate to the fast pace of the West, so different from the cotton fields of home. Yet he soon found a welcome diversion: a young actress by the name of Juliette Downs, the daughter of a prominent railroad executive, who looked past Rupert's lack of money and devotion to his work and saw a life of adventure traveling the globe alongside him. The pair wed in 1895, and not long afterward left for a posting in San Francisco, where they settled into a barrack on Angel Island. A winter rainstorm turned half of the island into mud, prompting Rupert to put Juliette up in a hotel in the city while he roughed it alone. For the first time in what would soon become a pattern in his life, he found his mind torn between his professional duty and concern about his young wife's increasing unhappiness as she faced the realities of a serviceman's life for which she was ill-prepared. His supervisors at Angel Island noticed that Blue's attention often seemed to be elsewhere. While he demonstrated diligence and tact on the job, he was still "somewhat disposed to be hurried," noted an officer in an early job evaluation.

Rupert was next transferred to Portland, Oregon, where to bring in extra money he took a side job as associate editor of the *Medical Sentinel*, a publication that billed itself as "The Local Journal of the Doctors of the Pacific Northwest." But even with a second source of income there was never enough cash at the end of the day. The pressure of supporting Juliette's tastes while also sending money home to his sisters and mother weighed heavily on his mind. "Ask mother if she can get along until May 30th or June 1 without a remittance," he wrote his sister Kate on yellow letterhead. "I promised Victor to send funds right away to her, but my finances are exceedingly low."

Only after a few years in the Service did he finally get an opportunity for adventure. In 1900, Rupert received an order to report to Rome, where he would be in charge of an investigation into rumors that plague was spreading through rural Italy. He jumped at the chance, undaunted by an assignment that could put him on the front lines of an epidemic. Juliette, meanwhile, could barely suppress her excitement at finally traveling to Europe, describing it in such alluring detail that her mother announced that she would be coming too.

After searching the Italian countryside for evidence of the disease, without result, Rupert spent his days strolling through Rome, drinking in its history. He paced along cobblestones that were older than any building he had seen back home and watched the sunset dance along the dome of St. Peter's Basilica. Through her family connections, Juliette secured a private audience with Pope Leo XIII. Rupert was not quite sure what to do with himself while in the man's presence, being neither Catholic nor understanding the French and Italian words the Pope spoke. Yet he felt calmed by the Pope's touch, a reminder of the fatherly affection that he was too proud to admit he missed. "I tease Juliette by saying that he liked me best as he took my head and face in his hands twice (blessing first,

benediction last) and only conferred this favor upon her once," he wrote in a letter home. "I believe he has blessed mother in her far away home, and for that he has quite won me."

The couple spent weeks touring Europe, giving Rupert his first taste of life outside of the United States. They visited London and Scotland and then arrived in Paris, where they were among the fifty million visitors to the World's Fair, delighting in a demonstration of the first-ever talking film. Just as he began to feel comfortable abroad, Rupert was ordered to Milwaukee, where he would be put in charge of monitoring illness among the shipping fleet on the Great Lakes. The return to the demanding reality of the Marine Hospital Service made the summer seem a dream. Money was still too tight, the Milwaukee winter too dreary. By the time Rupert and Juliette boarded a train to San Francisco the following year for his new assignment combating plague, their marriage was showing deep cracks. As the couple sped toward California, Rupert looked forward to the chance to start again.

White put him to work as soon as he reached the city, giving him day-to-day charge of the sanitation campaign in Chinatown, which allowed White more time to devise ways to pressure the Chinese Six Companies into revealing the plague victims he was certain were hiding in the district, rendering the cleanup effort useless. Unable to find allies on the state Board of Health, White turned to the police department, asking officers to alert him if they came across any Chinese who appeared ill during their periodic raids of Chinatown's gambling halls. When that proved unsuccessful, White asked Secret Service agents to trail Chinese residents in hopes that one would lead them to infected family members. He then posted agents at the Ferry Building, aiming to stop the flow of infected Chinese that he believed were being ferried across the bay to Oakland. "You cannot form any idea in Washington of the difficulties," White complained in a letter to Wyman.

With White's attention elsewhere, Blue was free to explore Chinatown at his own pace. He was impossible to miss as he roamed through the district, with his black hair, blue eyes and brawny build, towering over nearly everyone he passed. While he kept one eye out for areas that cleanup crews needed to address, he spent the majority of his time making idle conversation with Chinese residents, the first time that an officer in the Marine Hospital Service had attempted to forge a personal connection. His genial nature seemed to broadcast the sense that he was trustworthy, and he soon opened doors that had long been closed to other white doctors. In his first week, he discovered cellars filled with years of accumulated sewage and the decaying bodies of rats. While investigating an alley behind an upscale store on Dupont Street, he came upon more than 150 pounds of rotting meat lying in the open, overrun by the squirming bodies of rats and swarmed by insects.

White soon found himself drawn to a man who was so easy to like. Blue's "work to date has been most excellent," he wrote in a letter to Wyman, apologizing for his previous harsh assessment of the man. "The impression [that] he was not a man of pronounced personality and executive ability, although a very nice gentleman, is utterly erroneous. He has untangled a good many rather difficult snarls; has an immense amount of self-possession and good temper, and is altogether fully capable of acting as executive officer." White quickly realized that in Blue he had found a man who could deflect Governor Gage from undermining the Marine Hospital Service's mission. When the governor once again threatened to end the sanitation effort in Chinatown, White sent Blue to meet with him. After one lunch the governor came away mollified, as Blue had promised that Gage could send a doctor of his choosing to attend the autopsy of any suspected plague victim conducted by federal agents.

In San Francisco, Blue finally had found work that gave him a sense of purpose beyond a diversion from his crumbling marriage. Juliette, too, found reason to like the city outside of her husband's company. While Rupert waded through Chinatown's filth, she attended formal teas given in her honor at the mansions of San Francisco's high society, her father's wealth and prominence as a railroad executive her ticket into the city's social elite. "Mrs. Rupert Blue, what a beauty she is," noted the gossip column of the *San Francisco Call* after she was feted by more than fifty attendees at the Pacific Heights home of Mrs. Linda Bryan, then known as the grand matron of San Francisco society.

By June, Blue was promoted. Freeing the city from plague had become a futile task, in White's view, and he simply did not have the patience to preside over a long, slow defeat. He sent Wyman a telegram requesting a transfer and suggested that the Surgeon General appoint Blue in his place. Blue took over without ceremony, shouldering the twin responsibilities of sanitizing Chinatown and searching for additional victims of plague.

Over the following weeks, he began putting his fingerprints on the Service, shaping it to fit not only his own personality but his conception of what a doctor should be. Unlike Kinyoun, who was most comfortable in a laboratory removed from the complexities of human interaction, Blue thrived in situations where trust and tact were essential. That was not the only difference between the two men. Kinyoun paid an almost fanatical attention to rules, a natural trait in a man whose genius lay in following the complex procedures required by the science of bacteriology. Blue, whose academic work had been average at best, proved more willing to look at problems from multiple angles, searching for anything that might work, however unorthodox it might be.

One of his first moves after assuming command was to lease a small office in an alley off Chinatown's Portsmouth Square. There, in a two-room space that cost $75 a month, he set up a makeshift laboratory and morgue, finally providing the Marine Hospital Service with an outpost in Chinatown itself, rather than the distant Angel Island. Then, to solve the issue of bodies disappearing from the district before they could be examined, he convinced Wyman to allot him $35 a month to spend on establishing his own hearse service. He soon had a driver who could be sent with a horse and cart to any building in Chinatown as soon as a body was reported. The cadaver would be transported back to Blue's new laboratory, where it could be examined before anyone had a chance to hide it.

When state health officials protested, Blue revealed that underneath his genial nature lay a defiant streak. Unafraid of the repercussions of going against his promise to the governor, he issued a blanket ban that excluded state health officials from autopsies conducted on Marine Hospital Service grounds and instated a rule that no one except for federal health officers could enter the facility without his approval. Blue dismissed complaints by state doctors, writing in a private letter to Wyman that "we can bear a great deal more for the good of the Service and the cause."

His real first test came one evening in early July. As Blue and his fellow officers were concluding an autopsy in the small lab off Portsmouth Square, relieved by the absence of obvious plague bacilli in the body, they received a tip of a possible outbreak at the Yoshiwara House, a brothel at 845 Washington Street in Chinatown. Three of the seven prostitutes working at the establishment had developed large, painful buboes on their groins six days earlier and now lay nearly comatose with fever. The women had all lived in the city for about a year, making it impossible for them to have brought the disease with them. When Blue arrived, police officers were encircling the house, forming a quarantine line. Fearful of what the officers would do, a twenty-four-year-old prostitute by the name of Fuku Inaki, who had yet to develop any symptoms of disease, managed to slip away and flee to a house at 526 Pine Street, where she remained in hiding.

Blue and his officers pushed into the building and began evaluating the women, all of whom appeared near death. A bacteriologist drew blood samples from each woman and conducted a field test known as an agglutination reaction, which, though not as conclusive as Kinyoun's preferred method of animal inoculation, had been used with some success in India as a rapid method of determining whether plague was likely. The result was "immediate and characteristic," Blue wrote, noting that he was "absolutely certain that the three suffered from the same disease and this disease was bubonic plague."

There was nothing the doctors could do to save the lives of its victims. T. Shina Takagi, age twenty-three, and Miyo Ikea, age twenty-six, both died around three in the morning on July 9. Their bodies were taken to the Marine Hospital Service morgue. Federal doctors clad in rubber aprons conducted autopsies and took tissue samples from the buboes swelling on their legs. Cultures soon confirmed the presence of plague. Blue wired the coded message "Bumpkin malleate" to Wyman in Washington, informing him that two more verified cases were at hand. He sent another coded message two days later after Fuku Inaki, the woman who had escaped the quarantine of the brothel, was found dead despite having received a dose of the Haffkine serum from a Western doctor who treated her while in hiding. An autopsy revealed plague and syphilis. Federal doctors continued to monitor the remaining women in the brothel, expecting that they, too, would develop signs of the disease and die. Instead, health officials watched in amazement as Ume Kawamura, a twenty-two-year-old who was among the three initial cases, slowly began to recover, becoming the first patient followed by Marine Hospital Service doctors to survive the disease. None of the other women in the building contracted the plague, their lives untouched as if the disease had been satiated and lost interest.

As evidence piled up that plague was still in Chinatown, Blue felt himself getting boxed in. He had no appetite for trying to institute another broad quarantine, and little reason to expect that Wyman would support him even if he wanted to. With the situation more dangerous than anything Kinyoun had experienced, Blue realized how little official power he had. Marine Hospital Service officers learned that the three prostitutes who had died from plague had collectively had sex with at least fifty men—including several who lived outside Chinatown—in the days before their buboes appeared, expanding the zone of potential victims beyond the bay. Local newspapers, meanwhile, refused to give any attention to the latest outbreak, preserving the false sense of security that blanketed the city and left it all the more at risk. Even if the disease spread to white neighborhoods, neither residents nor their doctors knew what signs to look for, prolonging the time before federal doctors could come in and prevent plague from finding its next victim.

Blue continued to work in the shadows, hoping that luck would finally turn his way. He and his men injected themselves regularly with doses of the Haffkine serum, leaving them swaying between bouts of feverish delirium as they tried to solve a puzzle that could save countless lives. When no new cases were discovered in the following weeks, Blue began to question whether the Chinese were becoming increasingly skilled at hiding bodies or if there was another force at work preventing plague from exploding into the general population. The city's newspapers had lost interest in the Marine Hospital Service's efforts to fight the disease following Kinyoun's transfer, giving Blue the room to work out a solution away from the spotlight. Still, he could not help but worry that once again he would fail to measure up to standard and spent longer and longer hours in his small office in Chinatown while his relationship with Juliette withered.

His childhood insecurities rushed back that August when Victor arrived in San Francisco on a transport ship from the Philippines. "Of all the heroes with the late war with Spain, there is none that made a better record than Blue and none that wears his hard-won honors more modestly," wrote the *San Francisco Call*, a paper that had yet to mention Rupert's work in the city. When Rupert met Victor at the docks, his brother seemed to forget who he was, sending Rupert into deeper chasms of self-doubt. Victor later blamed his memory failure on an affliction that he called Phillippinitis. "When my brother met me this afternoon it was only when I heard somebody say, 'That's Rupert Blue, he used to be quarantine officer' that I remembered his name," Victor said to a reporter, adding that "about a dozen" soldiers on the ship home suffered from similar

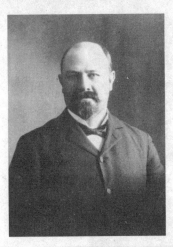

Joseph Kinyoun, shortly before he arrived in San Francisco. *U.S. National Library of Medicine*

Hospital Cove at Angel Island, which became Kinyoun's plague headquarters. *U.S. National Library of Medicine*

Chinese immigrants, such as these pictured in an illustration from *Harper's*, faced widespread bigotry in San Francisco. *U.S. National Library of Medicine*

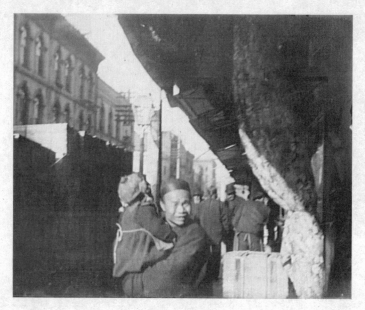

Fearing what white health authorities would do, residents of Chinatown resorted to hiding their children during the quarantines. *National Archives*

Men sporting long, braided ponytails known as queues—symbols of loyalty to the Qing dynasty—were common in Chinatown. *National Archives*

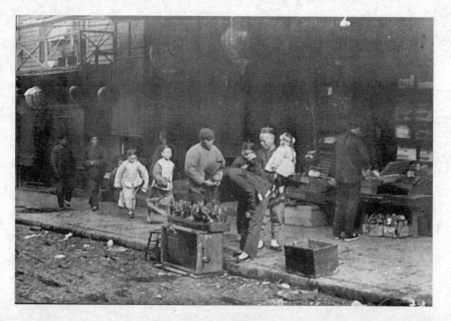

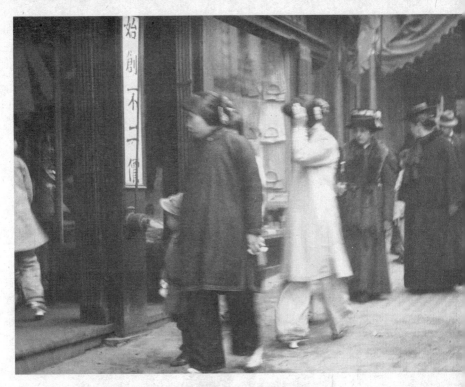

Chinatown's reputation for foreignness and vice made it a popular tourist destination. Here, white women and men take a daylight tour of the district. *National Archives*

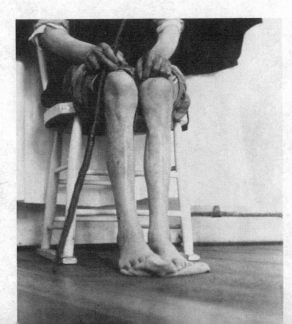

The hands and legs of a plague victim, displaying the characteristic black splotches that gave the medieval Black Death its name. *U.S. National Library of Medicine*

Rupert Blue, who twice saved San Francisco from plague. *U.S. National Library of Medicine*

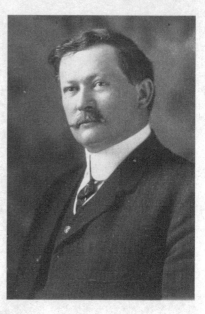

Health officers at a makeshift laboratory sliced open more than 100,000 rats, looking for signs of plague. *U.S. National Library of Medicine*

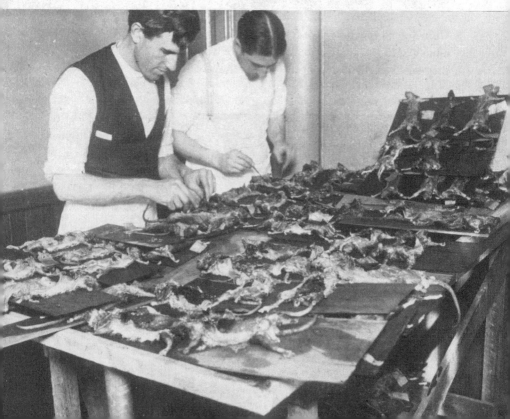

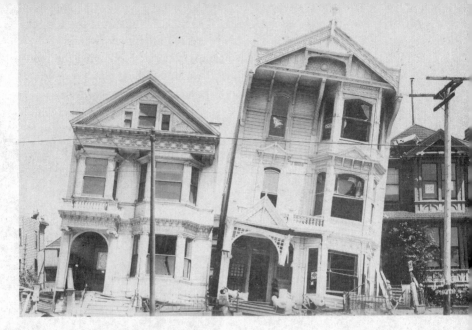

Over 80 percent of San Francisco's population was left homeless after the 1906 earthquake as apartment buildings and houses sank into the ground. *National Archives*

Some six billion bricks fell in the 1906 earthquake. For weeks afterward, the city was inundated with scavengers sifting through the rubble. *National Archives*

The Army erected more than twenty refugee camps in the city following the 1906 earthquake, including these tents set up in Golden Gate Park. *National Archives*

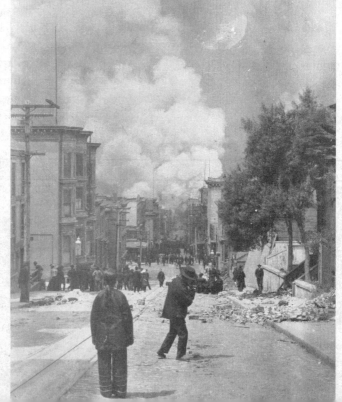

Residents of Chinatown watch as smoke billows over downtown San Francisco after the 1906 earthquake. *National Archives*

Rupert Blue (left) and Colby Rucker survey the damage to the city while searching for plague during the 1907 outbreak. *U.S. National Library of Medicine*

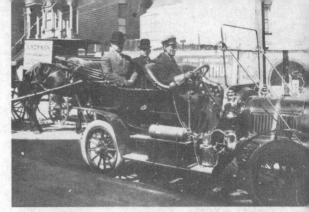

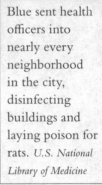

Blue sent health officers into nearly every neighborhood in the city, disinfecting buildings and laying poison for rats. *U.S. National Library of Medicine*

Under Blue's command, health officers eradicated more than two million rats in San Francisco. Here, an inspector condemns a backyard shack harboring rodents. *U.S. National Library of Medicine*

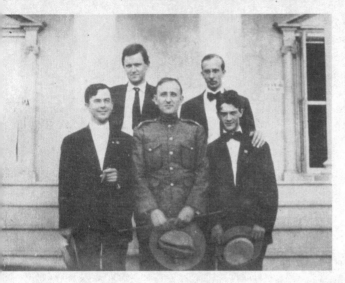

Dr. Colby Rucker (center) made dozens of speeches to groups across San Francisco, spreading the gospel of rat eradication.
U.S. National Library of Medicine

Rupert Blue (seated, center) and his corps of health officers who eradicated plague from San Francisco. To his left is Dr. Carroll Fox, who discovered that a quirk in the flea population prevented a wider outbreak. *U.S. National Library of Medicine*

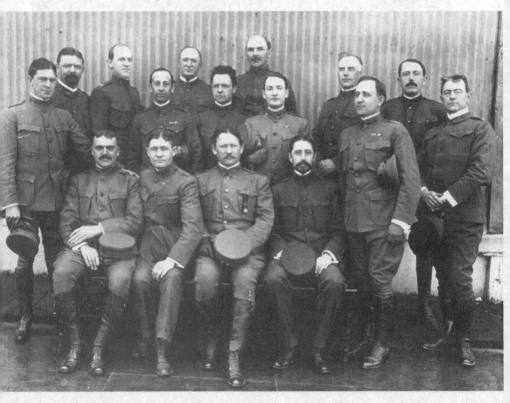

bouts of memory loss. Rupert entertained Victor and his wife for several days before they continued on to the East Coast, his damaged pride never recovering until Victor's train had receded from view.

The plague's apparent summer lull was broken just before Labor Day. The body of Lee Mon Chou, a forty-year-old man, was discovered one morning in the Oso Cigar Factory at 618 Dupont Street. The corpse was carted to Blue's morgue, where an autopsy revealed plague festering in the man's groin and right armpit. The roughly dozen men who worked alongside him vanished out of fear that they would be placed under quarantine or jailed, leaving Blue with no information about where the man lived, whether he had family, or where he might have traveled recently—anything, in short, that could help him save another person's life.

He had little time to investigate. Days after Lee's death, Juliette's father, P. L. Downs, was riding in a special first-class car when his train derailed and burst into flames in Montana, killing him and thirty-three others on board. Blue was granted an immediate leave from his post and took Juliette's hand as they boarded the next train north. Over the course of the three-day journey, Blue could only look back over the last months of his life with regret. His affable nature had helped smooth tensions between the Marine Hospital Service and the enemies that Kinyoun had made, but he could not point to any real progress. People were still dying, plague was still spreading and he was no closer to a solution. He knew that this was the greatest test he had yet faced, and his best and perhaps only chance to accomplish something that could rival the achievements of a brother whose fame had only grown.

As he looked out upon the Pacific, he vowed to himself that he would not fail.

CHAPTER 10

A MOST PECULIAR TEAM

Blue returned to San Francisco two weeks later without Juliette at his side. After nine separate postings in a span of seven years, their marriage could not weather any more upheaval. She remained in Washington with her mother, where she began the slow work of reassembling her life. Rupert, once more adrift, rode the train back down the coast alone, finally emerging in the San Francisco Ferry Building out of a late summer fog.

He had no place to go other than the tiny, two-room China-town laboratory, where a single radiator offered no match against the pervasive cold. Inside, vats of carbolic acid for use in autopsies inundated the office with a putrid smell that would seep into his clothes and cling to his mustache, reminding him wherever he went of his failures. Not that he was ready yet to experience life without Juliette by his side. The job was his only refuge and he immersed himself in the task of saving the city as a way to heal his own pain. He cleared all photos of Juliette from his desk, banishing anything that could trigger her memory, and posted a map on the wall above him, drawing a red cross at every address where a plague victim had been found. The grid of street lines became his sole focus. "Work of any kind, after such an experience, would [be] a blessing," he wrote in a letter to Wyman.

With his laboratory and morgue on the edge of Chinatown, Blue had established a closer physical connection to the district than any of his predecessors. Now he decided to take the next step and foster social relationships, too. He hired Wong Chung, a former secretary at the Chinese Six Companies, as an interpreter. Wong had worked for the plague commission earlier that year and was instrumental in helping the doctors uncover the first living patients to be officially observed. Yet after the plague commission doctors left his services had not been retained by Kinyoun or White, neither of whom could bring himself to believe that a Chinese person could be trustworthy. Blue offered Wong a rate of five dollars a week—equivalent to nearly $1,000 in today's dollars—and began treating him as a full member of his staff.

The sight of the two men standing next to each other—Blue a tall, muscular Southerner with a handlebar mustache and intense eyes, and Wong short, slight and bald except for the tightly braided queue of black hair dangling between his shoulders—seemed composed, as if arranged in an artist's study of contrasts. Yet the two soon developed a close bond, driven by their mutual mission. Blue chased plague as a way of finally winning the respect he had long sought and starting a new page in life; Wong, in turn, saw in the disease a chance to work with white officials as equals, united in the aim of saving the city they all loved. As he grew more comfortable with Wong, Blue began asking him to answer the questions that confused him about Chinese culture and its aversion toward medical procedures that could help combat an epidemic killing its own. Wong returned Blue's trust by bringing more cases of plague to his attention, certain that the federal doctor would not betray him or his people with another quarantine.

On September 11, 1901, Wong told Blue that Ng Chan, a twenty-eight-year-old clerk, lay close to death in the basement of the Fook

Lung grocery store at 821 Washington Street. Federal doctors who arrived at the building found fifteen other men living in the rank underground room, their small bunks partitioned by stacks of dirty boxes. Ng lay in a bed among them, overcome by a fever that topped 103 degrees. Doctors performed a quick examination of his body and discovered a swollen bubo on his right groin. Fearing plague, the men carried Ng to the nearby Tung Wah Dispensary, the closest thing to a hospital, and built a makeshift isolation ward while preparing to take a tissue sample that would confirm their suspicions.

That was as far as the doctors were able to get in treating a patient whom they believed carried a disease deadly enough to kill millions. The man's friends arrived at the facility and physically blocked the doctors from getting close enough to conduct any further procedures. The secretary of the state Board of Health then burst into the room and declared that the man was merely suffering from a venereal disease and must be released at once. When Blue refused, the official announced that he was taking command of the dispensary under a recently passed state law that granted the state Board of Health the authority to lift any locally imposed quarantine. Blue denied him again, objecting that treating a sick man in an improvised hospital bed could in no way be construed as a quarantine.

While Blue bickered over jurisdiction, Ng's friends formed a plan to sneak him out of the building to a ranch on the Sacramento River, where he could hide while his illness took its course. Wong picked up word of the plan from a janitor and alerted Blue. A police officer was posted at the man's door to prevent an escape. Ng remained in the care of federal doctors for three weeks and eventually recovered, though he continued to refuse tests to whether he had contracted plague. His survival gave the Chinese Six Companies exactly the case that it had been looking for. With evidence that federal doctors had insisted on a diagnosis of plague only to see the patient recover, Chinese patients in federal care began routinely refusing all medical tests, further complicating efforts to save their lives.

Yet the case proved to be a blessing for federal doctors despite their apparent failures. With Wong's help, Blue had successfully defused tensions between his men and Ng's friends and relatives, prompting the secretary of the Chinese Six Companies to offer unsolicited praise for the "pleasant and courteous manner" in which federal doctors treated the Chinese. Instead of seeing in Blue a reincarnation of the "wolf doctor" Kinyoun, the Chinese slowly began to believe that Western doctors were sincere in their desire to save lives. Federal agents, meanwhile, began to see in Chinese immigrants a people deserving of respect and humane care, a radical departure from the openly racist complaints of Kinyoun and White. "I do not think the Chinese here are very different from the human race elsewhere," one of Blue's subordinates wrote in a letter to Wyman. "And it is my conviction that if they are dealt with in a certain manner, the ends that sanitarians desire can be far more readily attained, and likewise with the Californians. My opinion is the result of five months of daily association and patient observation."

With Wong's help, federal doctors discovered the body of Tom Chin Fat, a thirty-five-year-old cook, in an empty apartment at 125 Waverly Place. Little about the man was known. Anyone who could offer information about his background or recent movements around the city had fled "like fleas before the body cools off," Blue wrote in a telegram to Wyman. An autopsy revealed swollen lymph nodes in the left groin and lower abdomen. Tests confirmed that they contained plague bacteria, making Fat the forty-second official victim of the disease in the span of twenty-one months.

The same day that Marine Hospital Service officials examined Fat's corpse, Alexander Winters, a fifty-year-old white sailor, arrived at San Francisco's Marine Hospital in the back of a horse-drawn cart. Though a sailor, Winters stayed close to home, ferrying schooners up and down the Sacramento River that brought goods ranging from bundles of hay to barrels of gunpowder into the city. The week before, he had suddenly begun vomiting while on a delivery run and run a high fever, which was followed by chills. He considered it nothing more than a bad flu until he came ashore in San Francisco and noticed a painful swelling in his right groin that made it difficult to walk. He checked into a room at the France House, a hostel at 149 Third Street then popular with sailors, and remained there as his condition worsened. After two days he fell into a stupor, and the men who shared his room took him to Marine Hospital. A tissue sample from the swelling in his leg revealed plague. Winters was placed in isolation, where he drifted in and out of consciousness, unable to give doctors any clues as to how he had contracted the disease.

Blue ordered his men to search for any connection between Winters and Chinatown, hoping to discover a link that would disprove his fear that the disease had again escaped the district. They combed through its brothels and opium dens for evidence that Winters had been there, yet found no links. "I would rather find a Chinese origin for this case, than to think that the sailors' haunts on the waterfront were infected," Blue wrote to Wyman, tempering his language so as not to reveal the full extent of his fears. "If we have then the two worst sections of the city infected, eradication of the disease is entirely out of the question, and the danger of an indefinite stay is enhanced."

Winters gradually recovered, confusing the doctors all the more. Thirteen days later, Marguerite Saggau, a fifty-three-year-old immigrant from Bavaria, died at the German Hospital. She had been admitted two days earlier after fainting in her room at the Hotel Europa, which was located one block north of Chinatown at 628 Broadway. Doctors initially suspected that she was suffering a uterine hemorrhage, until a full body examination revealed a large bubo on her right thigh. She was rushed to the isolation ward, where she died the following day. An autopsy and subsequent tests confirmed that she was the forty-fourth victim of plague, and the second white patient discovered with the disease in less than two weeks.

Blue again grasped for a connection to Chinatown, praying that the disease could still be contained. He took long walks around the dead woman's building, searching for clues that could connect her to the infected district down the hill, and traced all goods coming in and out of the Hotel Europa. He found nothing. The woman's husband and son remained healthy, ruling out infected laundry as the source, and no other occupants of the building developed symptoms. Once again, the disease had seemed content to select one victim and slink back into the shadows. He kept coming back to an idea that could explain how the disease was spreading, though Wyman had dismissed it before plague ever appeared in San Francisco. Yet Blue could not help but notice the possibility. The woman's home, he wrote in a letter to the Surgeon General, was only a few blocks away from Chinatown. That distance, he noted, was "a distance easily covered by rats in their migration."

The rat is the most common mammal in the world, living in close proximity to nearly every known human habitation. It seems designed on the principle that it must be ready for anything: it is an excellent swimmer, is blessed with a sense of smell that can detect poison in food down to the level of one part per million, and is equipped with teeth that are stronger than iron. Its skeleton can collapse, permitting it to fit through a hole the width of its skull. That level of mobility makes it an ideal urban dweller, able to enter and escape spaces that otherwise seem impenetrable.

Should it find its path on the surface blocked, a rat has two choices, both of them good. It can scale nearly vertical walls made out of every common material, and, once it nears the top, can jump more than four feet horizontally, allowing it nearly unlimited range in a city. Should it fall, it can easily survive a tumble from a height of up to 50 feet, roughly equivalent to the size of a five-story building. If climbing is not an option, then digging is: rats are known to dig dense underground labyrinths, as far as two feet below the surface, and are able to move swiftly through pitch-dark spaces by using their whiskers to guide them. Once introduced into a new environment, rats spread like a virus, their numbers expanded by a hyper fertility rate that can produce fifteen thousand descendants within a year from a single pair of rats. In environments densely laden with trash, rat populations can easily swell into the millions, making a significant die-off in their numbers unmissable by the human eye.

The link between a widespread die-off of rats and the arrival of plague has been obvious since antiquity, though the cause was uncertain. Ibn Sina, a Persian physician and philosopher whose eleventh-century tract *The Canon of Medicine* remains one of the most famous works in the history of science, noted that when plague was approaching, "mice and other animals which live underground fly from their holes and stagger from them like intoxicated animals." The Byzantine historian Nicephorus Gregoras, in describing an epidemic in Constantinople during the medieval pandemic of the Black Death, wrote, "The calamity did not destroy men only, but many animals living with and domesticated by men. I speak of dogs and horses and all the species of birds, even the rats that happened to live within the walls of the houses."

While Blue toyed with the idea that rats played a part in Marguerite Saggau's death, he had little scientific evidence to rest on. Medicine at the time largely considered plague a disease of filth, and had few conceptions of how it was transmitted from victim to victim. Paul-Louis Simond, a French researcher, had made a breakthrough discovery four years earlier, yet his finding was not yet widely accepted. Simond, inspired by the competition between Yersin and Kitasato to identify the plague bacillus, had travelled to Bombay in hopes of claiming the prize of discovering its mode of transmission. Doctors fighting the outbreak hypothesized that the disease spread through some sort of contact—whether inhalation, ingestion, or via open wounds on the body—with the urine or feces of infected humans or rats. Simond, who had studied intestinal parasites in Paris, came to doubt that theory. Instead, he noted, the bodies of patients treated at an early stage of the disease all exhibited a small blister that contained a mix of fluid and plague bacilli. These blisters—the size of an insect bite—were followed by the emergence of buboes in the lymph nodes in the groin, neck or armpits.

Convinced that insects were spreading plague through their bites, Simond went searching for what species was capable of transferring the disease not just from person to person, but from rat to rat. After first considering the cockroach, he turned his attention to fleas. The problem he faced was how to catch enough of them for use in experiments. When no other method of collection presented itself, he began dunking dead rats found in the homes of plague victims into a bin filled with soapy water, where he would rifle through their fur with his bare hands and pick out as many fleas as he could. When he examined the intestines of the insects under a microscope, he found that the fleas were saturated with plague bacilli.

The following year Simond tested his theory in Saigon with live rats he had caught in the homes of plague victims. He placed a flea-infested animal in a small metal cage that was not quite large enough for it to turn around in. Next to it he placed another cage of a similar size containing a healthy rat that had had no prior exposure to plague. Wire mesh walls and a thick layer of sand under each cage prevented contact between the animals and isolated their droppings. However, six-millimeter holes in the cages' screen allowed fleas to travel between them.

The rat taken from the home of a plague victim died on the second day of the experiment. Simond let its body sit for one additional day before removing it, giving fleas time to abandon the corpse and jump across the barrier to the still-healthy rat sitting nearby. An autopsy of the dead animal revealed an abundance of plague bacilli in the blood and organs. The healthy rat, now host to fleas from its dead neighbor, continued to eat normally for four more days, at which point it seemed to have difficulty moving. By the following evening it too was dead. An autopsy revealed plague bacilli in its kidney and liver. "That day, June 2, 1898, I felt an emotion that was inexpressible in the face of the thought that I had uncovered a secret that had tortured man since the appearance of plague in the world," Simond wrote.

His breakthrough was met with skepticism by his peers, who had trouble replicating his findings and remained moored to the notion that uncontained urine and feces were the primary vector of the disease. Surgeon General Wyman, in an article about the plague prior to its appearance in San Francisco, cast doubt on Simond's findings. "It is very possible that the fleas which infest rats, and which notoriously leave their bodies as soon as the cadavers become cold after death, may by their bites infect other rats," he wrote. Yet, he continued, "it is much more probable that the fleas or other insects having their habitat on animals deposit their dejecta, and in this way infect their bites." Instead of focusing on killing rats and their fleas to combat the disease, Wyman believed that doctors should work on cleaning up the soiled areas in which dead rats were discovered, largely through the copious application of boiling water. It wasn't until 1903 that French doctors working in Marseille proved that plague could not be transmitted among rats without the presence of fleas, confirming Simond's suspicion that the insect's bites had caused millions of deaths throughout history.

Though Blue was familiar with Simond's work, he did not have a chance to act upon his suspicions. The day after Saggau's death, the body of Lee Wing See, the forty-nine-year-old owner of a cigar factory, was found at 12 Spofford Alley. An autopsy revealed multiple buboes on his right groin and red and purple hemorrhagic spots across his arms, chest and abdomen. Two days later, the body of Chew Ban Yuen, a forty-year-old cook, was found at 109 Waverly Place, a building notorious as one of the worst tenements in the city. The man had recently arrived by steamship from Alaska, where he had worked in a cannery, though Marine Hospital Service officials could confirm no other details about his life as the two men who shared his room had vanished before federal doctors arrived. An autopsy found not only plague in the lymph nodes of his neck but tuberculosis in both lungs, a venereal wart and a streptococcal infection in his throat. The rotting corpse of Wo Tai, a fifty-year-old dock worker, was discovered on October 10, 1901, in the same Waverly Place building. A bubo bulged from his left groin. The following week, the bodies of two Chinese men were found in the neighboring building at 106 Waverly Place, both containing plague. The disease then retreated, as if it were biding its time. As winter set in, the number of new cases slowed to a trickle, leaving doctors wondering if it was dying out or hibernating to gather strength for the year ahead.

The cat-and-mouse game of the disease finally proved too much for Blue. Depleted by the months of failure both personal and professional, he wrote a personal letter to Wyman requesting a temporary transfer back to Milwaukee. It was not in his nature to run away from problems, he said, yet he simply could not go on. He needed something familiar, something that once again reminded him that he was good at some aspect of life, in order to rebuild his pride after the shame of watching his marriage crumble and death spread under his watch while he was unable to stop it. Feeling always two steps behind the disease simply compounded his heartache, stirring in him a sense of fatalism that he had never before experienced. The people of San Francisco—from the mayor to the press to the Chinese immigrants most likely to be infected—refused to believe that they were in danger, and Blue no longer trusted that he could make a difference, nor had the energy to try to protect the city from its own arrogance.

"Only a widespread epidemic, one [people] could recognize for themselves, will change that," he wrote in a letter to Wyman.

Deflated, with all sense of self-worth lost, Blue boarded a train bound for the cold plains of the Midwest, hoping that the open spaces would help him heal.

CHAPTER II

AS SOON AS POSSIBLE

A short article in the *San Francisco Chronicle* in April of 1902 made Rupert Blue's pain public. Its headline alone, "Dr. Blue's Wife Secures Divorce," was enough to cause a minor scandal in his hometown of Marion, where the voluntary termination of a marriage was still rare. In her complaint, Juliette said that Rupert had failed to materially provide for her, adding another layer to his humiliation. Rupert had not seen Juliette since he left her family home in Washington, and soon learned that she was preparing to sail to Europe for the summer, no doubt intending to immerse herself in high society and the possibility of romance after the drudgery of life with him in the Marine Hospital Service. Rupert, now officially alone, remained in Milwaukee, where he braved a future that he had never imagined.

His entire life, he had measured himself by the example set by his older brother, Victor, and never before had he found himself falling so far behind. Victor was a war hero and married with two young children, all but completing the circle of expectations set out by the social codes of the South. Rupert was none of that, and now his shortcomings were laid bare for all to see. He retreated into his work, grasping on to the one link that remained between his vision of what his life would be and how it was actually turning out. On his better days, he forced himself to accept invitations to dances and cocktail parties thrown by members of Milwaukee's upper crust, if for no other reason than to keep his social skills from atrophying from disuse. On other days, he spent more and more time in the boxing ring, hoping his fists could do what his brain had not and pummel his problems away. As he stood in the ring with his gloves on, delivering and receiving blows, he felt as if his body was exorcising the shame of the last two years of failure. The spread of plague in San Francisco was never far from his mind, yet he had no energy to return to the city and allow another defeat to enter his life.

With Blue no longer there to open doors and smooth over disagreements, federal doctors felt their influence in the city weaken. City, state and federal health officers were in open conflict with one another, leaving a coordinated response impossible. Under guidance from Governor Gage, state health inspectors began refusing invitations to attend the autopsies of suspected plague victims and would then claim that federal doctors were conducting them in secret and lying about the results. All attempts to force state health officials to acknowledge the reality of the plague were blocked, ignored or disregarded. One state doctor, when reached by telephone at his office by Marine Hospital officers informing him of the planned autopsy of a plague victim, pretended to be one of his clerks and said that his supervisor was away on business. Federal doctors grew so suspicious that one official wrote to Wyman and asked if the Secret Service could investigate whether state health authorities were working with the Chinese Six Companies to secretly dispose of the bodies of Chinese plague victims. "I regret [to] suspect Dr. Stone of such rascality, but I believe that he is perfectly suitable to such work," he complained.

Doctors on the city's Board of Health, meanwhile, were more focused on politics than fighting disease. Eugene Schmitz, a thirty-seven-year-old violinist whose flowing black beard and good looks prompted the press to call him "Handsome Gene," had launched a campaign as a third-party candidate for mayor. Behind his unlikely entry into the race stood Abe Ruef, a lawyer who had once studied classical languages at Berkeley before rising to the head of the upstart Union Labor Party. Together, Schmitz and Ruef ran on a racist platform that promised to purge the city of its Chinese population and increase the power of labor unions. The message resonated with the white working class of San Francisco following a year of citywide strikes in which the outgoing mayor, James Phelan, provided police protection to workers who crossed picket lines. Schmitz soon edged out his better-funded challengers. Though he had no governing experience, the new mayor leaned heavily on Ruef, who was widely considered the true mayor of the city. Together they began installing the most corrupt administration yet seen in the city, requiring bribes and kickbacks at nearly every level of government.

Schmitz diverted attention by rekindling anger at the plague campaign. In his inaugural address in January of 1902, the mayor singled out the city's Board of Health as one of the evils threatening the livelihood of working men in San Francisco and promised to hold its members responsible for "foisting upon the world sensational and ill-founded reports about the existence of bubonic plague in our midst." Two months later, he announced that he was removing four members of the board, including its lone bacteriologist, and maintained that he was "unalterably convinced" that plague "had never existed in the city." When a judge ruled that Schmitz did not have the power to fire board members until their terms expired at the end of the year, the mayor retaliated by slashing its funding so far that it could do little more than issue death certificates. His lone appointment to the board—a physician who also happened to be a significant campaign contributor—never showed up for meetings and instead spent a year traveling through Europe on the city's payroll, ostensibly to study the spread of infectious diseases there.

With all sanitary campaigns in the city suspended, there was nothing to prevent plague from spreading at will. The arrival of warm spring weather brought a surge of new cases. On May 25, the body of Chin Kee, a twenty-year-old bill collector who worked at the Horn Hong Newspaper Company, was found at his home at 811 Jackson Street. Tissue samples collected by federal doctors from a bubo in his armpit tested positive for plague. Four days later, Hong Quai, Chin's four-year-old nephew, died while being hidden from federal doctors in a coffin shop at 742 Pacific Street. Animals inoculated with tissue from the young boy's body soon died from plague, confirming the disease.

Four more bodies infected with plague were found in July, including two on the same block of Jackson Street, bringing the total number of cases confirmed by federal doctors since the start of the outbreak to sixty-one. The bodies of another nine victims were found in August, straining the ability of the bare-bones federal staff in the Chinatown morgue to keep up. Mark White, the doctor who had taken over from Blue, wired Wyman in Washington asking for an extra twenty-five dollars per month in his budget to spend on the supplies necessary to confirm each case of the disease. Wyman denied the request, hoping that the upswing would go away on its own.

The pace of death only quickened. On September 9, Chin Mong Yung Shee, a thirty-three-year-old woman, died in a small apartment at 40 Fish Alley after suffering from a high fever. An autopsy by federal doctors revealed a bubo on the right side of her neck. Interviews with men living in the alley revealed that two days earlier, a seventeen-year-old boy who lived with Chin Mong had also run a high fever, prompting his relatives to remove him from the apartment to avoid detection. He was taken across the bay to Oakland where he died three days later. No federal doctors were on hand to examine his body and no official cause of death was recorded.

Federal doctors only knew of the case—and the other twenty deaths from plague that had been confirmed so far that year—due to Wong Chung. Driven by his sense of purpose, the interpreter remained on the Marine Hospital Service payroll despite Blue's decision to transfer back to Milwaukee. He was among the few in San Francisco comfortable moving between the parallel worlds of Chinatown and the larger city and felt it his duty to save Chinese lives, even if that meant inviting in white doctors whose motives might not be always aligned with his own.

Still, the job took its toll. As he walked through the narrow alleyways of Chinatown probing for word of more victims, Wong struggled to keep at bay the inherent tensions in his life. By exposing the disease, he was increasing the likelihood that doctors would eventually find a way to end the epidemic. Yet he could not forget the fact that as a Chinese man he shared in the risk that each new victim he uncovered could be the one that finally prompted politicians to make good on their threats and burn the district to the ground. Though his identity pulled him in two directions, Wong knew that he was all that stood between plague and its future victims, and he was unwilling to allow the disease to kill in silence.

His work made him a marked man within his community. Not only was he working with untrusted white doctors, he served as a walking reminder that outsiders considered the district unfit for Chinese occupation and the Chinese an unwelcome part of American life. In April of 1902, to the cheers of white labor unions, President Theodore Roosevelt signed a bill that permanently banned Chinese immigration into the country. Those who were already in America were required to obtain a certificate of residency, and any Chinese immigrant found without the required papers was subject to immediate deportation. With no legal path for new arrivals into the district, San Francisco's business elite renewed its calls to relocate Chinatown from its central location. "The Chinese question is settled now. The labor elements have had their way, and Congress has renewed the Exclusion Act. There is no longer any use in keeping Chinatown as a sort of red herring to trail under the noses of visiting Congressmen" and frighten them into voting to ban Chinese immigration, wrote the influential *San Francisco News Letter* after more than 150 businessmen signed a petition calling on the mayor to resettle the Chinese in another part of the city. "The Chinese now have one of the best parts of town, and they have forfeited their right to it by their habits of life."

In the face of rising bigotry, the Chinese turned even more insu-
lar, seeking safety by having as few contacts with white San Francisco as possible. "We can save ourselves if we realize that we are all
in the same boat and will sink or sail together," argued the *Chinese
Western Daily* in an editorial. "Ruin will await if we behave like
fish that swim blindly into the boiling pot." Chinese tongs openly
patrolled the streets of the district, threatening anyone whose actions
brought unnecessary outside attention. With his work with the
federal plague doctors well known in Chinatown, Wong's friends
urged him to stop feeding information to the Marine Hospital Service if he valued his own safety. He refused their pleas and continued to alert the men at the Chinatown morgue to the location of
potential victims.

Wong could not remain safe for long. In early October, he
received an invitation to attend a special meeting of the Chinese Six
Companies, its exact purpose unspecified. He arrived at the organization's headquarters and entered the building just after sundown.
As he sat listening to the proceedings, unsure of his purpose there,
several gangsters rose from their seats and lunged at him. He fought
off the attackers and ran for the door, not knowing who else in the
room considered him an enemy. Only after the president of the Chinese Six Companies, for whom he had once worked as a secretary,
took him under his arm did Wong believe that he would escape the
building with his life. He watched as the men who had tried to kill
him fled, confirming his suspicions that the only thing uniting the
Chinese tongs and the white men in power was their willingness to
do anything to suppress the truth of plague in the district.

The attempt on Wong's life prompted Secretary of State John M.
Hay to warn the Chinese foreign minister in Washington that any
attack on Chinese residents working for the federal government
would be met by a decisive response. Undaunted by the attempt
on his life, Wong continued his search for victims. He soon alerted
federal doctors to the plague-infested body of Hoo Hing Bong, a
forty-seven-year-old man who lived at 743 Clay Street. He was the

eighteenth recorded victim of the disease in a span of two months, though the true number of fatalities was likely many times higher.

All the cases were found within a few blocks of one another in the northern half of Chinatown, suggesting that the disease was gathering strength. It was only a matter of time before it would begin spilling outward. As fall approached, federal doctors could only wonder if at last their nightmares had become real.

Wyman could no longer ignore the escalation of the disease, which was becoming a source of national embarrassment for the Marine Hospital Service. Federal doctors in San Francisco had battled the disease for three years and yet it only seemed to tighten its grasp. He ordered Arthur Glennan, a Marine Hospital surgeon then in charge of the quarantine station in Cuba, to report to California and inspect every city in the state with a significant Chinese population for the presence of plague, a group that included Fresno, Oakland, Berkeley, Stockton, San Diego, and Los Angeles. Before that, however, Wyman told Glennan to meet with Governor Gage, if for no other reason than to prevent another state challenge to his agency's federal authority.

Glennan arrived in mid-October and traveled to the Los Angeles suburb of Downey, where Governor Gage lived on a sprawling citrus ranch. Though he was still nominally in charge of the state, he was effectively without power after a series of embarrassing scandals—none of them related to plague—led Republicans to nominate another candidate in his place in the upcoming election. Gage had retreated to the citrus groves of Southern California to wait out the final months of his term and watched with growing resentment as an Oakland physician, George Pardee, secured the nomination that he considered his right.

Shunned by both Republicans and Democrats in the state, the governor welcomed the federal officer into his home and warmed to him once he offered a letter of introduction from Wyman. Yet he could not hide his anger once Glennan told him that California was once again facing a threat that Texas would quarantine all people and goods from the state on account of the persistent rumors of bubonic plague in San Francisco. "That god-damned plague again!" Gage bellowed. Not wanting to incite Gage further, Glennan said that the Surgeon General intended to address any cases found outside San Francisco as quietly as possible. The governor insisted that all of the supposed cases of plague were merely a form of syphilis, yet agreed to let Glennan conduct his tour of the state without obstacle. "I'll cooperate with Surgeon General Wyman and with you but damn the others," he told him. "Kinyoun would have been mobbed and hanged in San Francisco if I had not prevented it. And now, I am sorry that I did." As Glennan prepared to leave, Gage promised that he would "fix" newspapers in the state to avoid unwanted publicity. "This is the best that can be done at present," Glennan wrote in a telegram to Washington later that afternoon.

Two weeks later, state and local health boards from across the nation gathered for an annual meeting in New Haven, Connecticut. Though it was not on the agenda, San Francisco soon became the focus. City and state officials continued to deny the existence of the plague, while the Marine Hospital Service and national newspapers published details of the deaths of its victims. With officers from the Marine Hospital Service observing, the convention passed a resolution condemning California as a "disgrace" for its failure to readily share facts about an outbreak that was a "matter of grave national concern." A few health officials went further, arguing for a full quarantine of the state. Though the matter did not come to a vote, implicit in it was the charge that the Marine Hospital Service was not doing enough to protect the country from plague.

When confronted by health officials who lived outside California, Wyman downplayed the extent of the disease, aiming to spare the agency he considered an extension of himself from criticism. Pardee's victory in the gubernatorial race gave Wyman hope that with a physician in the governor's office he would have a closer ally in the state, allowing the Marine Hospital Service to do its work without harassment. Until he forged a relationship with the new governor, however, the Surgeon General continued to deflect any inquiries as to the true strength of the disease in the city. "The infection appears to be limited to Chinatown in San Francisco and to be restricted even within the limits of that locality to a very small area," Wyman wrote in a letter to Edmond Souchon, the president of Louisiana's state Board of Health, who was also one of the most prominent physicians in the South. "I was informed by the president of the City Board of Health, Dr. Williamson, that in his opinion there was very little of it."

Souchon had no way of knowing that federal doctors at the time were then examining the body of Deong Yuen Yum, a thirty-eight-year-old man who resided at 726 Pacific Street. An autopsy revealed plague bacilli in the lungs, abdomen and groin. The man's death made him the fortieth victim of the plague that year. Far from being contained, the disease was now accelerating its pace, bringing the city closer and closer to the widespread epidemic that had devastated Hong Kong. California, meanwhile, was no nearer to admitting the scale of the danger it faced. Gage, in his final message to the state legislature, once again blamed Kinyoun for sending what he called misleading reports about the disease, and cautioned the men standing before him that it was their duty to guard against any encroachment from the federal government.

Wyman sensed that he could not stall much longer. In mid-January, the health boards of eleven states met to address the issue of plague in California. The proceedings began with officials berating California's representative and shouting down his assurances that the incoming governor would implement all measures required to eradicate the disease, leaving him to later fume that he "was never treated with such discourtesy in my life." State health officials then turned their focus onto Wyman himself, peppering him with questions about the extent of the disease. Wyman would only allow that there was "not much" plague in the city, leaving conference members unimpressed.

A resolution was soon passed affirming that "the presence of plague in California was established beyond debate" and condemned Governor Gage and his state health board for obstruction. Given that the disease was entrenched in the city, the conference passed a second resolution asking the Secretary of War to relocate all troop transports from San Francisco to Seattle. If implemented, the measure would hollow out the economy of both San Francisco and the state. Its status as the most important port on the Pacific would crumble as national rail traffic shifted north, draining the power of the railroad barons who still effectively ran California.

The twin resolutions had little immediate effect. Newspapers in San Francisco called the measures "silly" and continued to downplay the idea that bacteriology was a valid branch of science. Instead, the city took the opportunity to congratulate itself. Thanks to "the persistent effort on the part of sober-minded San Franciscans [who] refute the baseless allegations of the men who attempt to make the world believe that it is necessary to use microscopes to discover an epidemic . . . this community has never for a moment been panic-stricken, as it might easily have become had the alarmist stories gone unchallenged," the *Chronicle* wrote in an editorial. Nor was the city's confidence that it could continue to deny the epidemic dented when health officials in Mazatlán, Mexico, blamed an outbreak of plague in that coastal city on a passenger arriving on a steamship from San Francisco. The Mexican government instituted a countrywide quarantine on goods and people coming from San Francisco, yet the city refused to believe it was true. Plague was somehow "an infectious disease which remains absolutely non-infectious in San Francisco but is capable, at the same time, of infecting persons down in Mazatlan," one prominent doctor joked to reporters.

Wyman, however, knew that his time was up. "It is absolutely necessary that confidence on the part of the health officers toward California authorities should be restored, and I am convinced that this cannot be done unless the governor in some manner acknowledges the presence of plague in Chinatown," he wrote in an urgent telegram to Glennan. "The situation is now entirely changed, and absolute frankness on the part of authorities of city and State is necessary to prevent pronounced hostile action, particularly when the conference of all the states meets in April." He sent another telegram to Glennan a few days later, suggesting that they bring back the only man who had seemed to make any real progress in the fight against the disease.

"Unless you wire me not needed will send Blue," Wyman wrote.

Glennan replied immediately: "Please send Blue as soon as possible."

CHAPTER 12

THE UNPLEASANT PAST

He was starting over yet again. As Blue packed up his home in Milwaukee, he intended to make a clean break this time. He cleared out every keepsake that reminded him of his life with Juliette, and sent boxes of books and clothing to his family in South Carolina with instructions to distribute them however they wished. Four months before his thirty-fifth birthday, an age by which most of his peers had families to support, Blue whittled his possessions down to what he could carry. After a year of wallowing in his pain, he was determined to leave it behind. Ahead of him was a new assignment, and with it the opportunity for redemption.

"I leave tomorrow for San Francisco," he wrote in a short letter to his sister Kate on January 31, 1903.

He reached the city a week later and checked into a small room at the Occidental Hotel. In the fourteen months that he had been away, plague had claimed another forty-one victims that federal doctors knew about, and countless others had likely vanished. The presence of the disease was no longer a local matter but an international scandal. British Columbia and Ecuador were now refusing all vessels from the state of California, and Texas, Louisiana and Maryland threatened to enact their own quarantines in retaliation for the city's stubborn refusal to acknowledge the crisis. Yet in the state itself, nothing seemed to have changed. Though he was a doctor by training, Governor Pardee rebuffed pressure from Wyman to issue a public statement admitting the existence of plague, a measure that would placate other states and give federal doctors more power. The newly sworn-in governor had narrowly defeated his opponent in the November election, and saw no reason to make enemies immediately in the state's largest city. All he would offer was a statement that he wished to work in "complete harmony" with federal officials, a declaration that no one outside California took seriously.

But Blue saw reasons for hope. If federal doctors could eliminate the source of the infection, they still had a shot at saving lives. And, for the first time in more than a year, politicians were willing to fund them. With the threat of a national quarantine becoming more real by the day, the city and state agreed to split the cost of cleaning up Chinatown, aiming to finally clear the district of its contamination.

Blue moved back into his old office at the edge of Chinatown and took charge of the largest sanitation campaign in San Francisco's history. Over the following weeks, he sent horse-drawn wagons carrying barrels of disinfectant up and down the district's cobblestone streets, spreading more than twenty-six thousand pounds of white lime powder that when picked up by the wind blowing off the bay looked like falling snow. State health officials wearing black bowler hats soaked the cellar of every building in Chinatown with carbolic acid and washed down the walls and floors with a solution of mercury bichloride and lye, leaving the neighborhood smelling like rotten eggs. Workers laid asphalt along Dupont Street, Chinatown's main thoroughfare, in order to allow the city's first street sweepers to motor down it three times a week.

After three years of failure, Blue knew that he had to do more than stage a short-lived cleanup. He sent inspectors, accompanied by interpreters, into each building, to record the number of apartments it contained and the health status of their occupants, providing federal doctors with the first accurate census of Chinatown and a rudimentary way to keep track of potential cases of plague. Officials took special note of subterranean passageways between adjoining structures, leaving some residents to suspect that it was the prelude to another quarantine. Though few denied the federal officials entry to their homes, all refused to give information about their neighbors. After years of abuse and distrust, the "Chinese race with few exceptions remained secretive and superstitious," Blue reported in a letter to Wyman.

Unlike Kinyoun, whose insistence upon total compliance from Chinatown's residents led him to escalate into ever more draconian responses, Blue remained measured. He had worked in the district long enough to accept that some of the hostility toward health officials was valid and that provoking further confrontation would only come back to harm him. Instead, he drew on his past. As a student, he had never been one to solve problems through a rigid adherence to formula, instead relying on a trial-and-error process that forced him to look for approaches that he might have missed. He accepted that a new situation was at hand. For three long years, federal doctors had demanded sanitation measures that had thus far proved ineffective at eradicating the disease. Perhaps, Blue thought, the problem wasn't the habits of the people in the district, as Kinyoun and Joseph White suspected. Perhaps it was something else.

Drawing on a suspicion he had first felt when confronted with the death of Marguerite Saggau in the Hotel Europa, Blue turned his attention to rodents, determined to discover whether the throngs of flea-infested rats that swarmed through the district—rather than simply filth or the foreign habits of the Chinese—were the true reason that the disease persisted. While Blue knew of Simond's work in proving the part that rats and their fleas play in spreading plague, no city had yet tried to act on it. He ordered his men to install hundreds of traps in Chinatown's sewers baited with arsenic-laden cheese. Autopsies were performed on the bodies of more than three hundred rats. None of the rats showed signs of plague in their lungs or buboes along their glands. Yet Blue was not deterred. His willingness to try new ideas—even when those notions clashed with the entrenched beliefs of his superiors in the Marine Hospital Service—had long been his greatest skill, and he leaned heavily on that openness at the time of his greatest need.

It was the first time in American history that a federal health officer had focused on killing rats as a way to combat a crisis. Cities across the country were becoming more sanitary, though rat eradication was often considered a side effect of those efforts rather than the intent. With telegraphs and automobiles heralding in a new, modern era, public health officers saw an opportunity to refashion the daily lives of Americans, a process that historians would later dub the Great Sanitary Awakening. Health officials pressed for legislation that ranged from mandating the truthful labeling of drugs to regulating the number of occupants allowed in urban apartments to requiring the pasteurization of milk and cheese in order to reduce the number of deaths from tainted food. The greatest energy was directed at urban tenement districts such as Manhattan's Lower East Side and San Francisco's Chinatown, with social reformers calling for measures such as adequate ventilation in buildings and regular trash pickup on the streets. Through a combination of small measures, public health officials cut down on the number of preventable deaths from germs and other agents of filth, allowing Americans to live and thrive on a scale that was unimaginable a generation before.

"Under more perfect sanitary environments we live longer, we live better; our energies, physical and mental, are stronger, and better fit us for entering upon a higher plane of living," Wyman once said in a speech that laid out the philosophy of the Marine Hospital Service to create what he called "slum-less" cities. "There is better opportunity for greater culture and refinement, greater familiarity with the higher laws of life, greater ability to comprehend our spiritual being and wrest from the unknown those higher principles of existence towards which we are now groping with unexplained instinct."

Blue directed the sanitation effort toward the specific goal of eliminating disease, largely by targeting the environments that allowed
rats to multiply. He instituted new rules that focused more on the
lives of rats than on the human residents of Chinatown. Dilapidated
balconies, rotting planks of wood, and makeshift additions to buildings were torn down throughout the district in order to eliminate
places for rodents to nest. Soon sunshine began filtering down into
the district's narrow alleyways, eliminating the persistent smell of
musk. The additional natural light proved to have unexpected benefits. Not only was sunlight a deterrent to rats, which have an innate
fear of bright light, but, as researchers were just then learning, the
plague bacterium can be killed by ultraviolet light alone.

There were some complaints about the destruction of buildings
that in some cases had stood for more than a decade, yet the anger
never exploded into a riot. Aware of calls among business leaders in
San Francisco to raze all of Chinatown and build a park in its place,
many residents assisted in the process of tearing down ramshackle
buildings, hoping that cooperation would allow the neighborhood
to survive. "Unless we clean the streets of Chinatown and deny
Caucasian men all their excuses, Chinatown's relocation is inevitable," the *Chinese Western Daily* warned.

Health officials discovered the first new plague victim six weeks
after Blue arrived, underscoring the reality that a simple cleanup
would not be enough to ensure the city's survival. The body
of A. I. Minegishi, a twenty-one-year-old Japanese woman, was
found at 520 Dupont Street. An autopsy uncovered black splotches
throughout her left groin, though no buboes. Tissue samples, however, revealed extensive plague bacilli, making her the first victim
identified by federal health officials in three months. Blue grew
convinced that more were surely to come. The dry summer months
lay ahead, a time of year when rats were known to leave their nests
in search of new sources of food and new mates. He redoubled his
efforts, praying that he could eliminate as many rodents as possible
before the breeding season.

He instituted a policy that he called "building out" plague, which for the first time required landlords to take responsibility for the ways in which their properties contributed to the spread of disease. Blue directed his attention first to rat-infested cellars along Fish Alley and the blocks surrounding the Jackson Street Theater. Landlords were ordered to pour a layer of concrete on their cellars or ground floors, which often sat on nothing but packed earth and offered a warm, dry place for rodents to build nests. Superstitious workmen burned the first foot of soil beneath each building, influenced by rumors prevalent since the medieval era that the plague infected the ground itself. Blue ordered broken drains fixed, cesspools filled in and any holes in a building's walls patched. Property owners who did not immediately comply were warned that the city would happily demolish the structure instead.

Nearly two hundred wooden buildings in the district were destroyed, with modern brick and concrete structures rising in their place. Stacks of discarded wood lay on the streets, remnants of the razed buildings. Blue barely noticed as the lumber slowly disappeared, claimed by scavengers for firewood. After three years of defeat, he was finally seeing progress.

Pietro Spadafora, a thirty-five-year-old Italian man who worked at the Southern Pacific railyards, was among those who often returned home with bundles of wood he had lugged back from Chinatown. Each morning he crossed the district on the way from his building at 19 Jasper Place in the Latin Quarter—a neighborhood home to a mix of Italian, Portuguese, French and Mexican immigrants now known as North Beach—to his job south of Market Street. Each evening he made his way back along the same path, picking up inexpensive fruit and vegetables from Chinese merchants. Like countless other Italian immigrants in San Francisco, Spadafora made enough money to keep his family alive, though just barely. Items discarded in the street were often given a second life in the Spadafora household, freeing up money to be used for another necessity.

One night Spadafora opened the door with planks of wood he'd

found in Chinatown tucked under his arm. He laid them in a corner and sat down to dinner with his wife, mother and two small
children. A few days later he developed a high fever and collapsed.
An ambulance carted him to the Southern Pacific Railroad Hospital on Mission Street, where doctors were shocked to discover a
swollen dark bubo in his right groin. He was put in isolation and
given an injection of the anti-plague serum, though doctors held
little hope that it would save him. He died the following day and an
autopsy confirmed the presence of plague, making him the ninety-
seventh known victim of the outbreak. Alarmed at the discovery of
a plague victim outside Chinatown, health authorities raced to the
dead man's home on Jasper Street, where they discovered his sixty-
year-old mother, Pietra, near death. She died the following day,
and an autopsy confirmed that she was the ninety-eighth victim of
the disease.

Blue questioned how plague had made its way from Chinatown
to the Spadafora household. He could only conclude that the discarded wood must have been swarming with plague-infested fleas,
which bit both Pietro and his mother. Fearing that other scavengers would spread the disease, Blue ordered that all debris from
demolished buildings in Chinatown be disinfected with a coating of
powdered lime, rendering it useless as firewood. He then instituted
daily health inspections of the Latin Quarter, determined to find
any other victims before the disease claimed another neighborhood
of the city.

It was through his continued focus on fleas that Blue left the racist
philosophies of Kinyoun and other Marine Hospital Service officials
fully behind. Kinyoun, for all of his laboratory brilliance, never let
go of his racial bigotry and remained convinced until the end that
the Chinese were an enemy that should be feared and distrusted.
Blue, never the best student or a natural leader, proved more willing
to trust what he saw before him and follow it wherever it led. The
sudden deaths of an otherwise healthy Italian man and his mother
proved that a conception of the plague as a racial disease was fool-

hardy and that skin color was no protection against a bacterium that seemed hungry to kill.

While careful to avoid the attention of newspapers and cause a citywide panic, Blue began concentrating more of his efforts on the Latin Quarter. He sent health inspectors into apartment buildings where no Asian resident had ever lived and demanded the same rat-proofing measures be put in place as in Chinatown. Concrete was poured along the floors of basements, while drains and debris were cleared and closed off, eliminating potential homes for rats. Blue hired additional men to serve as rat-trappers, laying poisoned traps throughout Chinatown and the Latin Quarter.

The Chinatown laboratory became a makeshift poison factory, where federal doctors brewed batch after batch of what was known as the Danysz virus. Named after its discover, a Polish researcher named Jean Danysz, the active ingredient was a strain of salmonella found to be lethal in mice and rats but harmless to humans and most other animals. Rats able to survive initial exposure to the virus soon develop immunity, however, making it a powerful but short-lived weapon. Blue's assistants became ever more adept at killing rats, slowly discovering what foods the rodents would take and how to avoid scaring them off. They soon learned that the Danysz virus was a fast-acting poison, often killing rats within a few steps of the feeding site. Aiming to use rats' scavenging methods against them, Blue's men also laced meat and fish with slower poisons such as arsenic, hoping that an animal would bring the tainted food back to its nest and infect others as well.

In order to expand his reach, Blue began offering a bounty of ten cents for every rat, living or dead, that was brought to the Chinatown laboratory. Each one was nailed to a roof shingle and autopsied before being tossed into a metal garbage can and incinerated. Governor Pardee, encouraged by the response, announced that the state would match the bounty. In his weekly dispatches to Wyman, Blue now included the number of rats inspected in his laboratory and how many had tested positive for plague. As the number of dead rats grew higher, he felt the first hints of progress, knowing that every rodent he eliminated from the city's streets was one less host for infected fleas.

No new human victims of plague were identified by federal doctors until August 10, when Charles Bock, a thirty-three-year-old blacksmith, died at the German Hospital on Noe and 14th Street. Bock had lived in the tiny village of Pacheco, located about thirty miles east of the city in the rolling hills of Contra Costa County. He had complained of a high fever that no medicine was able to dent, eventually prompting his brother to bring him to San Francisco to seek care. By the time he was admitted to the hospital, Bock had fallen into a semi-conscious state. He struggled to describe his pain to doctors, getting only so far as to report a feeling of dullness in his lungs. He died later that day, and an autopsy revealed a body consumed by the disease. Plague bacteria were found in the muscles of both his arms, his chest, abdomen, lungs, liver and spleen. Further tests showed that at the time of his death he was suffering from bubonic plague that had morphed into the highly contagious pneumonic form, making him one of the greatest threats to the city that federal doctors had encountered since the outbreak began nearly four years earlier.

His brother told federal doctors that Bock had not set foot in San Francisco since the Fourth of July, which meant that he must have been infected elsewhere. Health officials fanned out from Bock's farm in the village of Pacheco, searching for other victims. They found nothing, leaving Blue mystified. Then, on September 13, a thirty-one-year-old Canadian bridge builder named E. T. Slater died at the Southern Pacific Hospital on Mission Street. Slater, who had lived in the Contra Costa County hamlet of Danville, was admitted with a high fever and an examination revealed a dark bubo in his armpit. After his death, an autopsy confirmed that he too was a victim of plague, making him the 102nd death overall. Investigators learned Slater had last been in San Francisco in mid-August. He had only traveled as far as the plaza outside of the Ferry Building before returning to Oakland, leaving scant opportunity for him to have contracted the disease from a flea in the city.

Though the disease was still not contained in Chinatown, Blue turned his attention toward the rural expanse of the East Bay. Hearing rumors of a massive die-off of squirrels on several farms in Contra Costa County, he traveled out to the area intent on finding evidence for himself. Laboratory studies had demonstrated that, like rats, squirrels can become infected with the disease through the bites of contaminated fleas, though no scientist at the time had found a naturally occurring case of plague in North America. He made his way on horseback along dirt roads until he reached the small ranches where the two recent plague victims had lived. The terrain—rolling fields of green crops, where the only sounds came from farm animals—felt a world away from the claustrophobic squalor of Chinatown.

But finding dead rodents proved impossible. Blue learned that coyotes snagged most of them quickly, and those that did not die in the open perished underground in their nests. After struggling to find trappers willing to catch squirrels for him, he returned to San Francisco. As he sat in the saddle on his way back to the city, Blue could not help but feel increasingly uneasy, unable to shake the sense that his failures were compounding.

Over the following weeks, no new victims emerged in Contra Costa County. Blue resumed his focus on Chinatown, where, though the district was noticeably cleaner, the plague continued to linger. Four victims of plague were discovered in October of 1904, each one brought to the attention of federal doctors through the work of the interpreter Wong Chung. The following month, federal doctors identified three more cases. Among them were Slick Hat and Chew Soo, two seven-year-old girls who lived in buildings one block apart on Washington Street and were most likely friends. Federal doctors first examined Slick Hat after her mother alerted them to the girl's high fever and dark marks on her body, yet the disease was so far advanced that there was nothing they could do. After the girl's death on November 4, bacteriological tests confirmed plague. Three days after her death, her friend Chew Soo died in her family's apartment, another victim of the disease.

Blue could not make sense of the pattern of the epidemic, which seemed to strike several patients at once and then disappear. Doctors found no additional victims in December, only to discover three cases in January after a nearly two-month lapse. The victims all died within four days, frustrating Blue's ability to understand the disease or his own progress. "The appearance at this time of three suspicious cases was a surprise and a matter of regret," Blue wrote in a letter to Wyman. "I presume they are the result of the dry weather we have had since December 21st." He dutifully added red crosses to mark the addresses of the most recent victims on the map that hung above his desk. Fellow health officers would often catch him staring at the map as he tried to will himself into sensing a pattern that could point to the next victim before it was too late.

He always felt one step behind. Irene Rossi, an eighteen-year-old Italian immigrant, stopped showing up at her job at the Woods Clothing Factory, located at 27 Geary Street, during the first week of February. Her absence would have likely gone unnoticed had not another young woman by the name of Katie Cuka fainted on the factory floor and developed a suspicious swelling in her groin, prompting federal health officials to investigate. A federal inspector arrived and requested the attendance log for the week. When the foreman on duty checked his weekly sick list, he spotted Rossi's prolonged absence. He gave them the girl's address, and inspectors quickly covered the mile to the Rossi household at 6 Varennes Street.

They arrived to find the girl's parents, Luisa and Giuseppe Rossi, clad in black and planning their daughter's funeral. Over the last week, they learned, the young woman had developed a high fever and incapacitating headaches that kept her from leaving her bed. In her final hours, she coughed up a mixture of blood and foam that stained her teeth a deep red. With her parents unable to help, she died from what they believed was a severe case of pneumonia.

The doctors suspected plague. With as much tact as they could manage, they requested permission to examine the young woman's body and conduct an autopsy to determine the cause of death. Her father immediately refused. The doctors persisted, telling the grieving man that the procedure was required for all suspicious cases and could help prevent the same tragedy from falling upon another family's daughter. Rossi relented, but insisted on two conditions. First, the procedure must be done that night so that the funeral could take place the next day as planned. And second, he demanded to be present so that he could ensure that no undue harm would come to Irene's body. That night, he sat with tears in his eyes as he watched federal doctors at the Chinatown laboratory make incisions in his daughter's body and remove tissue from the lungs and spleen. Lab results revealed that she had contracted pneumonic plague, the most virulent form of the disease, which is spread by coughing. Had she left the house, she could have easily infected anyone who came too near.

Her family was not spared. Giuseppe died two days later at home and an autopsy revealed extensive plague in his lungs. The man's grief had masked his illness, even to himself. Doctors then conducted a frantic search for his wife, Luisa, who had vanished from the Rossi home after her husband's death. Two days later, a doctor in the Richmond District informed them that a patient was exhibiting signs of plague. Federal officials discovered Luisa hiding in her brother's home, burning with fever. She was immediately given doses of the Haffkine serum and admitted to the isolation ward at City and County Hospital. She died there from plague on February 19, 1904, making her the 118th victim of the outbreak.

The death of a white family outside Chinatown from the most virulent form of the disease forced Blue to question whether his focus on rats had simply made the situation worse. There were now noticeably fewer rodents in Chinatown, but Blue feared that his strategy of building out plague had prodded infected rats to migrate outside the district, bringing death with them. Blue wired Wyman to demand a rush shipment of two hundred additional bottles of anti-plague serum, though he hoped they would not be needed. Federal inspectors went door to door throughout the Latin Quarter, trying to identify anyone who had come into contact with the Rossis in the days leading up to their deaths. Health officials carried all clothing and furniture out of the Rossi home at 6 Varennes Street into the street and lit a massive bonfire, then fumigated the building with sulfur and lime to kill any bacteria that remained.

Haunted by the idea that the Latin Quarter could become as infected as Chinatown, Blue ordered additional inspections of every building in the neighborhood, with a focus on rats. After a demolition crew discovered the bodies of eighty-two dead rats lodged in the walls of a Chinese restaurant in the neighborhood, Blue directed his officers to place bait laced with the Danysz virus in warehouses, stables and restaurants throughout the district to remove easy sources of food. Dead rats soon began piling up in the basements of apartment buildings and along the sewer lines. The bodies were gathered up by either health officials or scavengers who brought them to the Chinatown laboratory to collect their bounty. Marine Health Service agents resumed the grim process of slicing open each one and looking for signs of plague, desperate for any information about a disease that they could not rein in.

After a week passed without new victims, Blue's fears of an outbreak of pneumonic plague subsided and he allowed himself once again to have faith that he was making progress. "I believe we have seen last of the pneumonic cases to be expected from the infection at No. 6 Varennes Street in the Rossi family," he wrote to Wyman. In the wake of the Rossis' deaths, Blue began receiving unexpected calls from white doctors alerting him to suspicious cases among their patients. "I am unable to decide whether these recent cases among the whites represent an increase, or whether they are the result of a desire on the part of physicians to openly diagnose plague," Blue confided to Wyman. "It would appear from conversations we have had with some of them, that they had had such cases before, but were not willing to make the diagnosis."

The sudden willingness of white physicians to admit that they, too, had treated cases of plague confirmed Blue's fear that the disease had been spreading secretly throughout the city. Yet he welcomed the help. He expanded the rat-proofing campaign further by ordering landlords in the Latin Quarter to demolish old wooden structures and replace them with buildings made of brick and steel. One week passed without any new victims, and then another, and another. Soon, Blue could point to the first three-month break between confirmed victims in more than a year. As the number of plague-free months climbed, Blue discovered that the city's overall death rate had fallen by 15 percent from the year before, a drop that he believed was in large part due to the work of his men in eliminating hundreds of thousands of rats from the streets and sewers. The effect was so pronounced that visitors who returned to the city after a long absence could talk about little other than its new, modern, sanitary appearance.

Four months after Irene Rossi's death, federal doctors had still not come upon any new victims, the longest lag between cases since the epidemic began. At six months, city officials began voicing the opinion that the presence of federal doctors and their expensive rat-trapping program were no longer needed. "The long interval that has occurred is considered by some of the people here to warrant the claim of extirpation of the disease," Blue wrote to Wyman. But he remained wary. "If by the beginning of the rainy season no case has occurred, then we may speak more confidently of eradication."

His worry was not just San Francisco. Two weeks after Irene Rossi's death, a thirty-nine-year-old Hispanic woman whose name was recorded only as Mrs. Frank Soto had died near Concord, a farming town in Contra Costa County not far from the homes of the two plague victims the year before. A local doctor alerted federal officials to the case. With the help of the coroner's office, Blue's agents secured samples of tissue from the dead woman's armpit despite protests of family members who resented the implication that she had contracted plague, which was still widely seen as a disease carried by filthy foreigners.

Frank Soto told doctors that his wife had not left the area around their home in months. An inspection of the ranch revealed no obvious sources of infection, though Blue did learn that a number of dead rats had been found in the stable, a sign that they could have been diseased. Still, the question remained of how an infected flea could have made its way from San Francisco to a remote valley in the East Bay. Blue could point only to the fact that the Soto home was located less than ten miles away from Port Costa, the main destination for sugar shipments from Hawaii. Though he had no way of proving it, it was possible that plague-infested rats had come ashore and spread their fleas to the local squirrel population, which carried it deeper into the countryside, bypassing San Francisco entirely.

Blue sent more agents to catch and examine wild rodents in Contra Costa County, with little success. A month after Mrs. Soto's death, federal officials learned that a young boy had died from what appeared to be plague. He and his brother had been hunting squirrels in the canyons near the town of Moraga and then cooked and ate their kill. A few days later, he developed a high fever and died in the family home. There was no way to determine the cause of the boy's death, however, as his body had already been embalmed and buried without an autopsy.

Blue wrote to Wyman to warn that plague-stricken rodents could soon infect the entire state, with their "burrows forming a continuous chain from one end to the other." Wyman agreed that the threat was serious and dispatched an officer to conduct a "complete and quiet investigation" of the state, armed with steel traps and a microscope to examine the bodies of any squirrels he could find. Blue, however, would not be a part of the operation.

The long break between plague cases in San Francisco convinced Wyman that the city was safe. In early 1905, he sent a short telegram informing Blue that he was being transferred to Norfolk, Virginia, where he would become the chief medical officer for the Jamestown Exposition, which was scheduled to open on April 26, 1907, marking the three-hundredth anniversary of the landing of the first permanent English colony in the Americas. The event was expected to draw visitors from across the globe, making any outbreak of illness at the event a national embarrassment to the Marine Health Service, to which Congress had given the responsibility of ensuring its safety. Wyman did not trust anyone other than Blue to handle such a high-profile assignment. Until construction began on the exposition, Blue would treat sick and injured sailors in Norfolk, a return to the more routine life of a Marine Hospital surgeon.

With Blue's transfer, most of the anti-plague measures in San Francisco wound down. The chief concerns of the city had shifted to quality-of-life issues—a sign of Blue's success. In Chinatown, the most persistent problem seemed to be residents' refusal to comply with rules against drying fish on ropes strung across the street. To mark Blue's departure, the city health department drew up a proclamation offering its thanks "to Dr. Rupert Blue for his skillful and energetic cooperation in all pertaining to the welfare of San Francisco's high sanitary state and commercial prosperity." Since the first known case of the outbreak in 1900, plague had infected 121 confirmed victims in San Francisco and the surrounding area and caused 113 deaths. As the spring of 1905 unfolded, San Francisco could look at itself and see a cleaner, modern city barreling into the new century. Blue, too, welcomed what the future would bring. Shortly after he arrived in Norfolk, he attended a large wedding, where he marinated in the accents and food of his native South. As he looked around the guests, he felt something that he had not felt in a long time: joy.

"The girls are very pretty and stylish withal," he wrote in a letter to his sister Kate. "Perhaps I shall meet my fate among them. You see, I have forgotten the unpleasant past."

CHAPTER 13

FOR GOD'S SAKE, SEND FOOD

At the age of thirty-three, Enrico Caruso was already considered one of the greatest operatic tenors in history. He had been born into a poor family in Naples, Italy, and received no musical training beyond singing in his parish choir until the age of eighteen. Within the first ten years of his career, he appeared on stages before packed audiences in Monte Carlo and London, and soon made his way to New York, where he became the chief draw of the Metropolitan Opera Company. His arrival in San Francisco in April of 1906 as part of the company's national tour was heralded by its newspapers as a coup for the city, providing yet another sign that it had outgrown its rough Gold Rush past and was truly becoming the refined "Paris of the West" that it claimed to be.

Lines formed outside the Grand Opera House on Mission Street when season tickets went on sale, with the cheapest package going for the equivalent of nearly $900 in today's dollars. Those who saw Caruso perform were quick to offer praise, and the avalanche of compliments began to leave the impression that San Francisco was keen to recognize not only Caruso's innate abilities, but itself for being able to attract such a talent. After his performance as Don José in a production of *Carmen* on April 17, Blanche Partington, the prominent music critic of the *San Francisco Call*, wrote that "*Carmen* rechristened itself for San Francisco last night . . . Caruso is the magician."

Caruso fell asleep that night in a suite in the Palace Hotel, the applause no doubt still echoing in his head. He woke shortly after 5:12 the next morning to the strange sensation that his room was swaying, as if on a ship in rough seas. Believing it at first to be a dream that he was on a steamer heading back to his home country, he lay still for several moments, waiting for the sensation to pass. Finally, as plaster started falling from the ceiling, he made his way to the window and opened the shade, wondering what it could be.

"What I see makes me tremble with fear. I see the buildings toppling over, big pieces of masonry falling, and from the street below I hear the cries and screams of men and women and children," he later wrote. "I remain speechless, thinking that I am in some dreadful nightmare, and for something like forty seconds I stand while the buildings fall . . . and during that forty seconds I think of forty thousand different things. All that I have ever done in my life passes before me."

From his window, Caruso watched as the greatest earthquake to hit San Francisco since its founding leveled the city. Men and women scrambled for safety as the ground porpoised and shook for forty-two seconds, each tick of the clock feeling like an eternity. Brick and glass showered down from buildings as power lines snapped and fell, writhing and hissing like angry snakes. By the time the ground stopped moving, more than thirty thousand buildings were gone. Clouds of dust hung low over the streets, blackening the air.

Those who were awake before the first jolt hit later claimed to have heard it coming, like the low rumble of a distant freight train in the dead of night. Thomas Jefferson Clark, a ticket clerk then on his way to his job at the Ferry Building, was walking along First Street when the earthquake struck. He was thrown flat on the ground, where the cobblestones around him "danced like corn in a popper," he would later say. He got up and ran down the middle of the street, fearing that he would be hit by falling debris. When he turned the corner of Market Street, he stopped short just before he fell into a hole more than five feet deep, where the pavement had simply disappeared.

Others died instantly when walls fell on them. On Howard Street, a firefighter by the name of James O'Neill was drawing water for horses when the American Hotel collapsed on top of him; on Mason Street, a police officer named Max Fenner died when bricks from an office building rained down onto his body. A few blocks away, the dome of the California Theater tumbled and crashed through the roof of a fire station next door, where Fire Chief Dennis T. Sullivan lived in a third-floor apartment with his wife, Margaret. Firefighters began frantically digging to free the Sullivans, assisted by reporters from the *San Francisco Bulletin*, whose office was across the street. By the time he was uncovered, the fire chief had a fractured skull, several broken ribs, a punctured lung, and lacerations on his right hip. His body was covered in burns from a radiator which he had been pinned against by the debris, leaving him near death. He and his wife were taken to different hospitals, and would never again see each other alive.

In the first minutes after the quake, deep fissures sliced through the cobblestone streets. The facades of buildings cleaved off and tumbled to the ground, revealing orderly rooms filled with furniture and bright wallpaper, as if the street were lined with enormous dollhouses. Homes that did not crumble buckled and slumped, leaving buildings leaning against one another like drunken friends. In other places, apartment buildings sank into the earth, trapping their occupants behind doors that would no longer open as water rushed in from cracked pipes. Straight sidewalks ran jagged; flat streets sported six-foot-high humps, as if a wave was frozen in stone. The force of the quake was so great that an engineer later exploring the fault line some thirty miles away discovered that the earth had jumped in some places by as much as seventeen feet and that the nearby mountains now stood four feet farther away. "If San Francisco had been at or near the fault line then there would not have been anything left of it," he later wrote.

The first major aftershock struck at 8:14, causing a second wave of panic. After the ground stopped shaking, hundreds of small fires erupted throughout the city. Water lines that had rumpled and split during the earthquake ran dry, leaving firefighters with nothing to counter the flames. Embers leapt from one building to the next, racing through entire neighborhoods and up the heights of downtown's greatest buildings. The magnitude of the fires created fierce winds, making downtown feel like it was in the middle of a hurricane. Great clouds of black smoke could be seen for miles, rising against the early morning sky. "The smoke began to curl up, and it curled up high and strong, for there had never been such a rich city in the history of the world—rich in rye and bourbon from Kentucky—rich in all brands in wine. Never before had there been a fire so richly fed," wrote Joaquin Miller, an aging poet and frontiersman, who watched the city burn from his home high in the Oakland hills.

Downtown the heat grew so intense that steel twisted and turned, popping the rails of the city's streetcar lines out of their beds and curling them up like elephants' trunks. Flames poured out of the highest windows of the Call Building, its grand dome towering over the city like a beacon of death. A few blocks away, workers at the U.S. Mint rushed to save the building and the more than $300 million in gold bullion held inside. As soldiers surrounded it to prevent looting, fifty employees of the Mint attacked the flames, armed with water pumped from an artesian well that had once been dug beneath it. Men more accustomed to counting money than to rough labor stood on the roof holding hoses to spray water on the flames, while those on the second and third floors passed buckets of water down long lines, and poured them onto the blaze. A sudden shift in the wind engulfed them all in black smoke, temporarily making it as dark as night, before a second breeze allowed them to resume their fight. Red-hot cinders the size of hailstones battered the roof, toppling its chimneys and piling up in drifts more than two feet deep.

Firefighters turned to dynamite, praying that the rubble would create a break in the flames. Trumpets sounded outside condemned buildings, a signal that everyone inside had to leave or would be shot. Panicked residents, some in their pajamas and others still wearing formal attire from the night before, fled barefoot into the streets, not knowing whether another aftershock would come. Only later did they realize that the heat from the fire made the ground feel like a stovetop, leaving them scrambling for anything to put on their feet.

Merchants raced to their stores, trying to save what they could from the fire and looters. The owner of Bacigalupi and Sons, then the city's premier seller of phonographs, later recalled running to his store at the corner of 4th and Mission as the fire bore down on the block. The heat was so intense that he scorched his hand while trying to unlock the shop door. After thirty seconds of trying to pry his way in, he realized that the plate glass window lay shattered on the sidewalk and he climbed through the empty space. Soldiers shot a man attempting to rob Shreve & Co., then known as the most famous diamond jeweler on the West Coast, and left his body to burn in the street as a warning to others.

Crowds of dazed refugees, many still dusted by the white plaster that fell from their bedroom ceilings, trudged up the city's steep hills carrying whatever they had managed to save from their homes. One woman carried an empty birdcage with the bottom missing; another, only an umbrella. Overcome with shock, strangers sat down next to one another in the street and wordlessly watched the city burn below them. "Everywhere were trunks with across them lying their exhausted owners, men and women," Jack London later wrote in an article describing the city's devastation. "Often, after surmounting a heart-breaking hill, they would find another wall of flame advancing upon them at right angles and be compelled to change anew the line of their retreat . . . Here and there through the smoke, creeping warily under the shadows of tottering walls, emerged occasional men and women. It was like the meeting of the handful of survivors after the day of the end of the world."

Shortly after noon, Mayor Schmitz held an emergency meeting of staffers and prominent businessmen, if only to assert that the city was in fact still there. City Hall had collapsed, leaving only its ruined copula, so officials met in the nearby Hall of Records. Schmitz yelled as loud as he could, straining to make his voice heard over the sound of booming dynamite and debris crashing down outside. "Let it be given out that three men have already been shot down without mercy for looting," the mayor began. "Let it also be understood that the order has been given to all soldiers and policemen to do likewise without hesitation in the cases of any and all miscreants who may seek to take advantage of the city's awful misfortune." The building trembled from the force of an explosion nearby, and the police chief begged the mayor to leave before the structure collapsed. The meeting resumed in the middle of Portsmouth Square. Within hours, the Hall of Records would fall to the fire.

As the fires continued to burn, refugees overwhelmed the Ferry Building, where the clock on its gleaming white tower was stuck at the moment when the earthquake hit. Ferries, warships, and in some places rowboats clustered along the city's waterfront, picking up as many people fleeing the flames as they could. Patients from St. Mary's Hospital were loaded onto ferryboats after the building caught fire, with doctors and nurses carrying those too weak to walk. "If you picture the scenes described and imagine the horror a thousand times greater you will still know less than I have personally witnessed," George Bernard Musson, the captain of a British steamer that was at port in San Francisco and became a makeshift refugee camp, wrote in a letter home. "Motherless children and childless women are here, the old and aged and young are all here, high born and low are all one class." The city of Oakland sent fire engines, hoses and dynamite by ferry, taking thousands of scared men, women and children on the return voyage. Governor Pardee, when he learned of the devastation in the city, sent a telegraph to Los Angeles, begging "For God's sake, send food."

Those who could not reach the water fled to the parks. In the

Presidio, more than thirty-five thousand men and women crowded onto the golf course. Soldiers at the nearby U.S. Army base began issuing tents, blankets and tins of crackers as rations, along with cans of condensed milk to women carrying babies. Residents of Chinatown, hearing rumors that no provisions would be given to Asians, trudged to a windswept section of Golden Gate Park, where they ate whatever they had been able to salvage from their homes. Only after the poor treatment of the Chinese threatened the country's relationship with China did President Roosevelt direct the army to provide rations and shelter to all refugees, regardless of race. "President directs you furnish same shelter and camping facilities to Chinese as to others . . . use your own discretion as to whether special camps shall be established for them," wrote Robert Shaw Oliver, the acting Secretary of War, in a telegram to General Frederick Funston, who was in command of the Presidio.

The following day, engineers jerry-rigged systems that connected firehoses to intact sewage lines, finally giving firefighters something to use to beat back the flames. Sailors on Navy vessels that responded to the city's distress calls unfurled a mile-long hose from Fisherman's Wharf, providing a constant supply of seawater. Firefighters in Jackson Square used it to save the A. P. Hotaling warehouse, which at the time was the largest liquor repository on the West Coast. The accomplishment would later spur Charles Kellogg Field, a writer for *Sunset* magazine, to quip, "If, as they say, God spanked the town / For being over-frisky / Why did He burn His churches down / and spare Hotaling's whiskey?"

It took three days for the fires to burn themselves out. In neighborhoods where grand theaters and restaurants once stood lay only blackened ruins. After the flames subsided, the heat emanating from the toppled buildings remained so intense that men and women trying to return home fainted in the streets. Refugees crowded around any source of water, as if a desert oasis. A broken water main at the corner of Powell and Market gushing out cold seawater attracted a crowd of hundreds, who sat on the curb and bathed their singed feet in the stream flowing through the wreckage.

By the end of the week, more than 80 percent of San Francisco's buildings were destroyed, and more than 250,000 people were living in the city's parks. The Army oversaw twenty-one of the eventual twenty-six official refugee camps, with an isolated camp built for residents of Chinatown. In the Presidio, thousands of white tents were arranged in an enormous grid, where the paths between them were given street names. "The demands upon the medical department have been enormous," George Torney, the chief sanitary officer at the U.S. Army Hospital in the Presidio, wrote in a telegram to the Surgeon General of the Army in Washington. "The fire is evidently under control and the urgent problem is now one of sanitation."

On the other side of the country, Rupert Blue was occupied by the mundane task of conducting routine inspections of federal buildings in the nation's capital. When word of the earthquake and devastation reached Washington, he packed his belongings at once, knowing it was only a matter of time until he was called back into service in California. He received orders from Wyman on April 21 to proceed immediately to San Francisco and reached Oakland four days later. He rode a ferry into the devastated city the next morning, seeing nothing but ruins where a week earlier its skyline had stood. As he passed through the charred streets near the waterfront, he looked up and saw the shell of the Call Building standing like a monument in a graveyard. He soon reached Golden Gate Park, the home of the city's makeshift sanitation headquarters, and joined a meeting already in progress between state and city health officials, who were discussing how to save San Francisco from further ruin.

The danger from the earthquake and fires had passed; the chief concern now was disease. Rats were already overrunning the refugee camps, where discarded food lay rotting in plain sight. The stench of untreated human waste sitting in shallow, hand-dug holes wafted throughout the city on winds whipping off the bay. Without proper sanitation and clean drinking water, deadly diseases like cholera and typhoid were sure to spread, if they had not done so already. Already, twenty cases of smallpox had been identified in Oakland, where neighborhoods had been overrun by refugees from San Francisco. Governor Pardee asked Blue to take a ferry back across the bay and make an inspection of the camps holding some of the 150,000 estimated evacuees, a total which had doubled Oakland's population in less than a week,

Blue made his rounds the following day and was shocked at what he saw. "For the most part they consist of wooden shacks, hastily constructed in vacant lots, parks and in the suburbs of the city, and are supplied with shallow latrines, and open kitchens which offer no obstruction to the ingress and egress of flies," he wrote in a report to Washington. At Lake Merritt, near the city's downtown, he found two large camps and a smaller hospital camp for sick refugees nestled between them. Human waste saturated the ground, while rats darted in and out of tents. Fearing the spread of cholera from the open sewage, Blue disbanded the sick camp and sent its residents elsewhere. Over the course of the day, he toured camps holding an estimated 30,000 refugees, including four thousand Chinese whose numbers overwhelmed the city's small Chinatown. His instructions at each step were the same: latrines must be dug deeper, screens installed to protect food from flies, and systems set up to collect trash and cart it away as quickly as possible—a protocol more often used to maintain sanitation in a war zone than in the heart of a major American city.

The next day, he returned to San Francisco, which health officials had divided into sections in order to make sense of the devastation. He was given the responsibility of salvaging a district bounded by Bay, Market, Valencia and Mission Streets, the most heavily damaged part of the city. "A rapid tour of inspection revealed a deplorable state of affairs with regard to sanitary measures for the protection of these people against disease," he wrote. More than 30,000 people were living in shacks and tents, while those whose homes remained standing were forced to cook in makeshift ovens in the street. No water or sewage connections remained intact, leaving a dwindling water supply and growing mounds of untreated sewage festering in uncovered pits swarming with flies. Public kitchens stood nearby, their food set out in the open as they prepared to serve meals to hundreds who lined up in city squares, a layout that seemed designed for contamination.

Already disease was spreading, especially in the informal camps that pocketed the ruins. "On Gavin Street there are two children with sore throats which appear suspicious of diphtheria," an Army medical officer reported. "There are about 100 families here with no shelter and no bedding whatsoever." Another forty-five people had congregated at the foot of Hyde Street, while the intersection of Stewart and Folsom was home to about sixty people, all without any shelter, bedding or ways to maintain hygiene in a place that had lost all of the sanitary infrastructure underlying the modern world.

Blue ordered the construction of large public toilets and had them connected to the few functioning sewer pipes that remained. Waste that could not be taken out of open-air pits was smothered with chloride of lime and carbolic acid before being buried. Realizing that refugees were hoarding food in their tents and attracting rats, he demanded that all cooking be done in communal kitchens, and installed screens to prevent flies from spoiling food left uncovered. Residents were ordered to collect their garbage into huge piles, which were burned hourly and carted away.

Slowly, the contours of a functioning city began to reemerge from the rubble. The U.S. Mint opened its doors and became San Francisco's only functioning financial institution, handling all relief funds that came into the city from the East Coast. Over the next several weeks, more than $40 million flowed through the Mint's doors, allowing homeowners to cash insurance checks and purchase the supplies needed to rebuild. Those whose homes were beyond repair were placed in temporary wooden cottages, which at their peak would house nearly seventeen thousand refugees who paid two dollars a month for their accommodations. "San Francisco is beginning to rise again out of its ashes," wrote Samuel Fortier, a professor at Berkeley, in a letter dated April 25. "There is no lack of confidence. The courage of the people is simply remarkable . . . the people of San Francisco seem determined to begin at once to build a new San Francisco, which will far surpass the old in every essential feature."

Despite Blue's fears, no major illnesses swept through San Francisco in the aftermath of the earthquake and fires, dispelled in part by the sanitary measures that he and Army medical officers implemented. Residents fortunate enough to return to their homes began moving out of the refugee camps in early May, allowing the choreography of daily life to begin anew. Confident that the danger of cholera and other diseases spread by sewage had passed, Blue turned his attention to plague, which he feared was still spreading in Contra Costa County.

He soon received word of a patient exhibiting strange symptoms in Oakland, and travelled across the bay to the home of Louis Scazzafava, an Italian teenager who had come down with a sudden high fever and dark, swollen glands on his thighs. Scazzafava told him that he had gone hiking with a friend in the hills just behind the University of California, Berkeley campus a few days before, where he had come into close contact with squirrels that seemed to be acting strangely. Tests revealed that the boy had contracted plague, the first confirmed case of the disease since Blue had left the city the year before. Scazzafava was placed in isolation and given an injection of the Haffkine anti-plague serum. Perhaps owing to the early treatment, he slowly began to recover.

Blue canvassed the Oakland and Berkeley hills, seeking information on anyone else who might have come down with the plague's telltale collection of symptoms. He found no one. The only conclusion he could reach was that the boy had the unfortunate luck to have encountered an infected squirrel, just as the plague victims in Contra Costa County had the year before. Plague-infected fleas were still lurking in the rolling green hills, and it would only take something as innocent as a teenager going for a hike for the disease to cross over into the human population.

Before he could investigate further, Blue received a telegram from Wyman directing him to return to Virginia and resume his duties at the Jamestown Exposition. He collected his small suitcase and boarded a train, but not before writing to Wyman to warn him that the plague appeared to be slipping out of San Francisco and into the East Bay. "There seems nothing more for me to do here," he cautioned, noting that the sanitation plan for the refugee camps of San Francisco was now in place. "Yet I am loath to leave in view of the possibility of plague among campers and picnic crowds in the Berkeley Hills."

As his train chugged out of Oakland and over the foothills of Contra Costa County toward the East Coast, Blue prayed that his fears were nothing more than worry, and that he would not have to return to San Francisco on another frightful mission.

TWO PERCENT

No one in San Francisco had time to rest. There was too much work to be done.

An estimated six billion bricks lay strewn throughout the city in the aftermath of the earthquake, leaving piles of rubble in some cases nearly as high as the buildings they had once been. In the first weeks of the cleanup, soldiers forced able-bodied men into teams and put them to work clearing streets and dumping bricks into the bay. Yet it was evident that San Francisco needed more help if it was ever going to become anything more than a remnant.

Within two weeks of the disaster, the ruined city had turned into a magnet for scavengers and tourists unable to resist the lure of destruction. Sightseeing wagons clopped through the devastation, gawking at families trying to recover what they could from their demolished homes. "I request you to let no morbid curiosity take you to the burnt districts, but be content to do your share toward bringing about conditions in which the past may be forgotten and the future made bright for the upbuilding of our city," wrote Mayor Schmitz in an open letter. Magazines published articles detailing how visitors could help the city and what they should avoid lest they become a hindrance. "It's all right to go to San Francisco if you can do some good there. Take with you a bottle of milk that you know is pure and sweet and fresh, or a package of condensed milk, or a suit of little baby clothes, if you have one that the baby has outgrown . . . Don't go to stand and gaze," noted an article in *Organized Labor*, the official magazine of the state's building trades council.

The city worried that investors on the East Coast, spooked by their unfamiliarity with earthquakes, would refuse to purchase the municipal bonds necessary to fund San Francisco's reconstruction and searched for ways to demonstrate that progress was already underway. City officials worked out of the partially destroyed City Hall, directing inspectors to evaluate every building still standing and flag those that required demolition. All available lumber, brick and glass in the state was put on trains heading toward San Francisco, along with men and women seeking work. The chief counsel of the Western Pacific Railroad wrote a letter to the mayor suggesting that "immediate steps should be taken to procure all unemployed carpenters, brickmasons and builders that can be obtained from the various cities in the United States." Railroads offered reduced rates for skilled workers from the Midwest and East Coast to travel west, where they were guaranteed a job.

Even at this low point, San Francisco could not shed its bigotry. The Pacific Trades Council and other construction unions in the city refused to work on buildings or sites cleared by Asians, requiring the mayor to intervene to prevent a riot. The mayor assured construction companies that "he could not countenance importation or use of Coolie labor in San Francisco nor would he favor competition of cheap foreign labor against American white labor," wrote William Howard Taft, then the Secretary of War, in a telegram to President Roosevelt three months after the earthquake.

Progress remained slow. More than forty thousand people were still living in refugee camps, and on the first anniversary of the quake two-thirds of residents lacked functional sewers. Empty lots throughout the city were littered with the remnants of destroyed roofs, broken-down ceilings, and scattered debris. Souvenir hunters

CHAPTER 14

and scavengers had picked over the ruins for everything of value. All that was left were mounds of trash and dust, the residue of a city in a hurry to right itself.

On May 27, 1907, thirteen months after the earthquake, a horse-drawn buggy pulled up outside the U.S. Marine Hospital in the Presidio. Inside lay the slumped body of a sailor named Oscar Tomei, burning with a high fever. Tomei had fallen into a coma before he could describe his pain, leaving doctors to strip off his clothes. They discovered a swollen bubo on his groin, which tested positive for plague. Faced with the first new case of the disease in three years, federal health officers raced to the waterfront, hoping to piece together how the man had contracted the disease.

He had worked aboard a tugboat named the *Wizard*, but beyond that everything about his life—where he lived in the city, his acquaintances and his recent whereabouts—remained a mystery. Nor could his former shipmates provide any clues. The *Wizard* had shipped out to sea shortly after discharging the sick man two days before, and sank off the coast of Mendocino with everyone aboard. Tomei died the afternoon he arrived at the hospital without regaining consciousness. With all information about the sudden reemergence of the disease lost, doctors could do nothing but wait and pray that it claimed no additional victims.

For ten weeks, they heard nothing. Then, on August 12, a twenty-one-year-old Russian sailor from the steamer *Samoa* named Alexander Ruvak died at the same hospital, from what appeared to be pneumonia. As medical staff prepared the death certificate, a doctor noticed suspicious dark lumps on the dead man's neck and called for an autopsy. Tests revealed that they were buboes, laden with plague bacteria. Federal doctors hurried to the *Samoa*, where they found dozens of dead rats, fleas and bedbugs but no other apparent human victims. The ship and its crew were ordered into quarantine at Angel Island.

While the *Samoa* was being towed to the island, a physician named Guido Cagliari called the city Board of Health to report suspicious symptoms in two of his patients who were now near death in their home at 20 Midway Avenue in the Latin Quarter. Doctors found Francisco Conti, an Italian immigrant who had worked the past nine months at the Musto Marble Works, lying semi-conscious with a fever. At his side was his wife, Ida Conti, who had arrived two months before from Italy, her temperature spiking at 104 degrees. Dark bulges protruded from their thighs. Health officials carted Francesco to the isolation ward at City and County Hospital, where he recovered over the following weeks. Ida died at home before doctors could move her. An examination of her body confirmed plague.

The following morning, Guadalupe Mendoza and Jose Hyman, two Spanish laborers who shared a shack on Pacific Street near the waterfront, were admitted to City and County Hospital, burning with fever. Both died that same afternoon. As their bodies were prepared for autopsy, a sixty-three-year-old orderly named Jeremiah O'Leary disposed of the dead men's clothing. O'Leary had an open wound on his hand, yet thought nothing of it as he went about his duties. Mendoza and Hyman both tested positive for plague. Not long after, O'Leary was admitted as a patient, with frighteningly similar symptoms. Terrified that he too would contract plague, an intern named Arthur Reinstein refused to treat O'Leary, who died two days later. Reinstein was dismissed for moral cowardice and dereliction of duty, but not before submitting a letter of resignation for what he called "obvious reasons."

With six victims in the span of less than a week, the plague had reappeared in the city, baffling health officials who could find no pattern among the dead. Chinatown, the center of the last outbreak, seemed to be the only neighborhood spared. Unable to focus their attention on a single neighborhood, health officials felt pulled in every direction, not knowing where the next victim might emerge. Even if they wanted to, there was no neighborhood to quarantine, no community to target, in hopes of walling off the disease. For the first time since plague appeared in the city seven years before, it felt like all of San Francisco was at risk.

Meanwhile, a forty-year-old Irish laborer named John Casey seemed to be getting sicker as he lay in his bed at City and County Hospital while recovering from a routine procedure. Doctors discovered plague-infested buboes swelling throughout his armpits and groin. Within days, a nurse and an intern at the hospital also fell ill and displayed the telltale mark of the disease. Inspectors looking for a cause of the outbreak canvassed the dilapidated hospital building, then widely considered among the city's worst. They found rodents everywhere, in numbers too staggering to count. "The rats have so many runways deep through the hospital and have burrowed so deep even under the soil; into the sills of the building," one health board member wrote after touring the facility. "The sewers are filled and the foundation is full of them. Sulphur does not penetrate sufficiently to destroy all the rats."

The hospital was placed under quarantine on August 27, less than two weeks after its first plague victims arrived. Patients who were free of the disease were taken to Laguna Honda, a small hospital which had opened in 1866 to treat Gold Rush prospectors and now survived as the city's largest almshouse. After that institution quickly filled up, patients were dispersed to hospitals throughout the city, filling so many beds that officials had no choice but to put some up in horse stables at the Ingleside racetrack. City health officers ordered an iron fence built around City and County Hospital to seal rats within the building while crews cleansed it with sulphur and carbolic acid. Construction crews refused to take the job, fearing that they too would come down with the deadly disease. Doctors on staff began working double shifts, first tending to their patients and then going outside to erect a wall they prayed would save the hospital and pin the plague inside.

Unlike during the previous outbreak, there was no denying the danger the city faced. Nearly all of the most recent victims were white, proving that the plague was not restricted along racial lines.

Its return came at a time when San Francisco, still struggling to restore the confidence of investors and tourists from back East, could least afford it, and spread with a ferocity never before seen in the city. Mayor Edward Taylor, a poet and lawyer then in his first weeks of office following a municipal corruption scandal that had ended with the arrest of Mayor Schmitz, telegraphed President Theodore Roosevelt at his summer home in Oyster Bay, Long Island, begging for help. Roosevelt assured the panicked mayor that the federal government would send its best men.

Rupert Blue, the only person in the country with a track record of successfully subduing plague, was unaware of the outbreak. After returning from San Francisco the year before, he had resumed his position as head of sanitation at the Jamestown Exposition, where his chief problem was a group of workers who had caught typhoid fever after drinking from wells that Blue had repeatedly warned them were tainted. Wyman telegraphed Blue to leave at once for San Francisco and take with him anyone he thought would be of assistance. Orders in hand, Blue gathered a team of doctors in Washington whom he considered among the service's finest, experienced in combating diseases including smallpox and yellow fever. Together, the men boarded a train on September 6, bound for the West Coast and the wide epidemic that Blue had long feared.

There was no time to lose. Plague was racing through the city, killing its victims with alarming speed. By the time that Blue and his men arrived in San Francisco on September 12, health officials had identified twenty-five cases since the start of August, with thirteen of them fatal. There seemed to be no pattern, no clues as to where it would strike next. One day, a clerk at an elegant hotel in Nob Hill fell dead after working his shift; the next, a man living on Harrison Street in the gritty South of Market neighborhood succumbed to the disease in his squalid apartment. Chinatown remained largely spared. The lone death in the district came when Chin Mon Way, the sixty-three-year-old president of the Chinese Six Companies, contracted the disease and died two days later, leaving his organization in disarray.

With many of the city's hotels still-charred ruins, Blue checked into the Little St. Francis, a makeshift wooden hostel built in the middle of Union Square. Rumors of his return to the city put San Francisco on edge, terrified at the prospect that he would institute a quarantine that would choke off its recovery. Hoping to project calm, Blue penned an open message to the residents of San Francisco, which was published in its newspapers. "To the People of San Francisco," he wrote. "Rumors of an alarming nature having reached the board of health in regard to bubonic plague, the president of the board, by its authority, hereby declares that there exists at present in San Francisco nothing that need cause any alarm, much less the quarantining of the city, and there is at present no intention to make such a quarantine . . . Every precaution is being taken by the federal authorities, in co-operation with the state and city boards of health to stamp out such of the disease as is here." In private, he knew that the situation was far more grave. "The campaign is likely to be a long one, and the infestation will be fifty times more difficult of eradication than before," he wrote in a letter to a colleague in Washington. "The foci are to be found all over the city, the greater number existing in the burned district where, on account of the protection afford by the ruins, the rats multiply in countless numbers."

Blue had no headquarters, nor laboratory, nor medical equipment, forcing him to improvise. With office space in the city still sparse, he rented a two-story Victorian house at 401 Fillmore Street which became headquarters for his team of twelve doctors. The city allotted an additional thirty-six sanitary inspectors and provided him a private car and driver, allowing him to motor through destroyed neighborhoods where streetcars still could not go. On his drives through the city, Blue felt the full weight of his task. The geography of the place—a roughly fifty-square-mile peninsula made up of hills and valleys, forests and sand dunes, densely packed neighborhoods and crowded stables—offered countless obstacles. In order to save San Francisco he would have to tame the nightmare scenario the Service had long known was possible: multiple sections of the city affected at once, with a rapidly rising death toll and nearly all of its victims white. The only thing that gave him hope was Chinatown, which even in the devastation stood out for the fact that it was the lone part of the city not teeming with rats, a fact he attributed to the poison and other measures he had put in place roughly two years before.

With the zone of infection now stretching over the full city, Blue designed a plan built around the still-radical idea that plague was a disease of rats that periodically crossed over into humans, and not the result of filth or foreignness. The virus festered in areas that afforded food and shelter to rats and their fleas, he believed, and not because of any inherent flaws in a victim's virtue or race. "Rat fleas bite men," Blue would later write. "They usually prefer to bite rats, but when the sick rat is dead and his eighty or eighty-five boarders have left his cold cadaver and camped for a few days without food, in a crack in the floor, or under the mould-board, or in a little inch of dust in a corner that the broom failed to reach, they will bite anything. They will bite a white man just as quick as a Chinaman, or a Hindu, if they can reach him."

In disease Blue recognized a shared human trait, and, for the first time since the plague epidemic began, he set about purging all of San Francisco of its rats without regard to human race or ethnicity. As in most cities, rodents were considered a natural part of the urban landscape and not a harbinger of disease. Rats were such an everyday part of city life that construction workers rebuilding office towers downtown would toss leftover food from their lunches into vacant lots, knowing that the rodents would clean up after them. "That was what rats were for," Blue would later write, describing the city's attitude. "Nobody had any objections. God made them scavengers, so let them scavenge." The ruins of the city provided

near-infinite nesting places, allowing the rat population to expand
without constraint. On his return to the city, Blue was struck by the
fact that fleas were "unusually prevalent," while "on account of the
great catastrophe sanitary conditions were unusually bad."

Drawing from his experience in the aftermath of the earthquake,
Blue divided the city into thirteen districts and unleashed teams of
ratcatchers into each one. At his prodding, the Merchant Association
sent letters to every address in town, urging residents to set out traps
and poison, seal their garbage in rat-proof containers, and seal every
rathole as soon as they saw it. Health inspectors would visit each
property twice, looking for rats. Clad in heavy pants, tall boots and
leather gloves, they clinched the cuffs of their pants around their legs
with string before entering a suspected area, aiming to give fleas no
exposed skin on which to bite. Inspectors would note the number
of rats taken from each location, the gender of each animal, the date
and whether the house had been visited before. Every afternoon,
teams arrived back at the Fillmore Street headquarters with their
hauls. Rats found alive were tossed into vats of boiling water, a tac-
tic meant to quickly kill fleas clinging to their bodies. Each carcass
was nailed to a wooden shingle and given a number along with a
short description of where it had been caught.

As the bodies of thousands of rats piled up inside the house, federal doctors wearing rubber gloves stood before long dissection
tables and sliced open the chest of each corpse, as if in a ghoulish
disassembly line. They peeled back the skin of the animal, to inspect
its glands and spleen, searching for inflammation and buboes that
suggested plague. When a rat appeared to have the disease, a bacteriologist plucked it from the line with metal tongs and took additional
tissue samples. After a culture was prepared, suspected plague cells
were injected into guinea pigs to confirm the diagnosis.

Soon, doctors were filling ten steel garbage cans a day with
splayed rat carcasses, which were then tossed into an incinerator.
The sheer number of rodents that passed through the building led
doctors to start referring to their headquarters as the Rattery. On

some days health officials would stop in amazement, wondering how it was possible for there to be this many rats not only in San Francisco but in the entire world. To protect themselves from the bite of an infected flea, the men took frequent doses of anti-plague serum, which, when combined with the rank smell of blood and dizzying amounts of formaldehyde, often left them barely able to stand.

No matter how many rats passed through the Rattery, the disease kept spreading, picking off victims as if by whim. In Noe Valley, five out of six members of a German family living in a well-kept row house succumbed to the plague, sparing only an eighteen-month-old boy. Health inspectors searching for the source of the infection tore up the wooden floors and discovered the bodies of nineteen plague-infested rats. Across town in the Marina District, eighteen residents of one of the largest remaining refugee camps died after contracting the disease. Among the dead were a five-year-old named Thomas Herrera and a sixteen-month-old toddler named Mary Costello, both of whom had lost their parents among the estimated three thousand who perished in the earthquake.

Blue walked through the camp, where more than two thousand refugees lived in tiny wooden cottages laid out in a grid atop of the former Lobos Square. Rats swarmed over the dreary grounds, building nests under the wooden sidewalks and feasting on garbage. The dense collection of people in temporary shelters made the widespread application of poison unfeasible, lest a child get its hands on tainted food left in a trap. Unable to see a solution, he ordered his men to catch as many rats as possible by hand and returned to the Rattery to search for an answer.

He had little time to think. In the Mission District, two young boys playing in an unused cellar discovered the corpse of a rat. Emulating their father, who was an undertaker, they performed a mock funeral service before picking up the animal and putting it into a shoebox as a casket. They dug a hole with their hands and buried the rat, completing the ritual. They then ran back to their home at 2888 Mission Street, unaware that their clothes were crawling with infected fleas.

A few days later, their thirty-seven-year-old father, Otis Bowers, fell ill with a high fever and debilitating fatigue. When he discovered a swollen lump on his right thigh his wife, Margaret, called a doctor, but it was too late. Otis lay dead within the hour. Two days later, doctors were again summoned to the house, where they found Margaret near death. They rushed her to the nearest hospital, where she was administered immense doses of the anti-plague serum. The medicine did not stop the disease, and she succumbed to what was later identified as pneumonic plague. Only then did the young Bowers boys think to tell federal doctors of their discovery in the cellar. Health inspectors dug up the rat they had buried and brought it to the Rattery at 401 Fillmore Street. An autopsy revealed internal organs bursting with plague.

The second-wave death toll reached sixty-five by December. Blue's men were catching and killing more than thirteen thousand rats a week, yet that seemed to barely dull the ferocity of the disease. Though few national newspapers had yet to report on the outbreak, Blue sensed that the window of time in which he could operate without bringing in unwanted attention was closing. Norway had declared a quarantine on goods or visitors arriving via San Francisco, and Blue feared that other states and countries would soon follow. His only hope was to double down on his campaign against the city's rodents, elevating rat-killing from an urban chore into something approaching a science. "Rats are extremely wary animals and enough cannot be caught by inexperienced men to greatly reduce their numbers," he later wrote. "It therefore becomes necessary to place intelligent men at this task and train them carefully in their duties. A man can no more be made into a rat-catcher by giving him a rat trap than he can become a soldier by being provided with a rifle."

Blue knew that even with dozens more paid ratcatchers San Francisco would not stand a chance against the disease. To eradicate plague, he would need the help of the city's residents. He directed his second in command, Colby Rucker, to write a primer called "How to Catch Rats" which drew from what Blue and his team had learned. The essay was circulated throughout the city, effectively deputizing each resident of San Francisco into Blue's corps.

"It is first to be remembered that the rat is a very wise animal and that the whole operation of trapping him is a test of wits between man and the rat," it began. Catching a rat required playing to the animal's natural curiosity and need for variety. Rodents living in slaughterhouses were easily enticed into traps by vegetables, while those which had made their nests near produce stands seemed to crave meat. Regardless of their immediate preferences, all rats appeared to be drawn to traps that included some mixture of fish heads, raw meat, cheese, fresh liver, fried bacon, pine nuts or carrots, Rucker wrote. The job was not finished once a rodent entered the trap, he added. When caught, a female rat should be left where it lay, as its cries would often attract nearby males and any of its offspring into the same lure. Finally, he wrote, do not kill rats where they were caught, as their squealing and the smell of their blood was known to frighten other rats away.

Writing circulars would only go so far, of course. The ethos of doing as one pleased in one's private life was as much a part of San Francisco as the fog and the hills, and the city had never before come together in a collective effort that required its residents to change their behavior. Even in the aftermath of the earthquake and fire, it was an accepted fact among its citizens that the city's resurrection was achieved mainly through individuals looking after their own interests, with the Army and government assistance programs only making it possible for the private market to operate. Not only that, but Blue knew that even with the rising death toll from the disease he faced a problem of scale. Coming on the heels of the near destruction of the city, an urgent call to clean up trash and trap rats in order to stop illness from spreading seemed pitifully small by comparison.

To fully get the public's help in killing rats, Blue would need the press. All of the city's newspapers had responded favorably to the ratcatching campaign, with the exception of its largest and most powerful publication, the *Chronicle*. Intent on getting the paper on his side, he requested a meeting with the paper's publisher and co-founder, Michael Henry de Young, a man who personified the city's freewheeling boomtown era that Blue's methodical approach to sanitation sought to end.

At the age of fifty-eight, de Young was a year older than the state of California itself. He had started what became the *Chronicle* with his older brother Charles at the age of sixteen after taking out a twenty-dollar loan from their landlord. As it grew, the paper helped shape the city as it transformed from frontier to metropolis, though the de Youngs could never quite leave the lawless past behind. In 1879, Charles shot and injured a mayoral candidate by the name of Issac Smith Kalloch because he suspected that the man was spreading rumors that de Young had grown up in a brothel. Kalloch recovered and went on to win the race. The following year, his son, seeking revenge, snuck into the *Chronicle* building and fired five shots at Charles from close range, killing him instantly. His one errant shot smashed through the window of Michael's office and cut a hole in the wall above his head. Five years later, Adolph Spreckels, one of the four sons of rival newspaper publisher Claus Spreckels, followed Michael de Young into the *Chronicle* building seeking revenge after de Young had accused his father of manipulating stock prices. Spreckels called out de Young's name and then fired at him with a pistol, hitting him in the left shoulder. He fired two more shots, one of which hit de Young in the arm and the other which lodged in a package of books that he had held up as a shield. Spreckels later pleaded not guilty to the crime by reason of temporary insanity and was acquitted after a six-week trial, with de Young's unpopularity widely suspected to be the chief reason for the court's leniency.

The experience only hardened Michael, who went by the profes-

sional name M. H. By the turn of the twentieth century, the power
he had accumulated as the owner of the largest paper in the largest
city on the Pacific made him one of the state's most important power
brokers, and he was unafraid of using his resources to further his
aims. The year before the plague reemerged, the *Chronicle* had put its
weight behind a local measure that forced Japanese students to attend
segregated public schools, with its editorial page calling all Japanese
immigrants who reached California "human waste material." The
policy turned San Francisco into a national embarrassment, with a
writer from *Harper's* calling it "probably the worst city for a boy to
grow up in that there was in the United States," though the city did
find support from Southern Democrats who feared federal intervention into their own segregated schools. Japan, which was emerging as a powerful force in the Pacific, lodged an official complaint
with the U.S. State Department over the school ban. Threats of
war receded only after President Roosevelt stood before Congress
and called the attempt at segregation a "wicked absurdity" and San
Francisco's leaders "infernal fools." When San Francisco still refused
to allow Japanese students to attend schools with white classmates,
Roosevelt brokered what was known as The Gentlemen's Agree-
ment, under which Japan would issue passports only to those going
to Hawaii, and the San Francisco school board rescinded its policy.

With the humiliation of federal intervention in city matters still
burning, de Young was outwardly dismissive of anything connected
to Washington, much less a thin federal health officer who was once
again raising the issue of plague. When Blue arrived, de Young
coldly motioned for him to enter and sat facing him in a stiff-backed
chair at the foot of an enormous fireplace, its redwood mantel decorated with carved vines.

Blue, by then adept at massaging the egos of powerful men, began
the conversation by asking for de Young's help in preventing a tragedy. By printing the truth of the reemergence of plague in the city
and the role of rats in spreading it, the paper could save the lives of
its readers and make de Young a hero, he said, hoping to appeal to

the man's vanity. While Blue talked, de Young remained impassive, finally saying that he would not commit to anything. The conversation clearly over, Blue thanked him for his time and left the building, gripped in the hot panic of failure, not knowing whether his overture had worsened the situation. De Young was "a strange, stubborn man and may turn his guns on us with greater effect than ever," he warned in a letter to Wyman.

He had no way of knowing whether he was making progress and yearned for some tangible evidence of victory. As the final days of 1907 ticked away, Blue could see only failure. Federal doctors had confirmed the deaths of seventy-three plague victims since August, and there was no sign that the disease was abating. Blue worked punishing hours in the laboratory at 401 Fillmore Street, often emerging not knowing whether it was morning or evening, a confusion only worsened as he stumbled through chilly clouds of fog that seemed to leach even the memory of warmth from his body. He drove his corps of ratcatchers to work longer and faster, and prayed that by the conclusion of each week he would have something to show for all of his work. With the push to trap and dissect as many rats as possible overwhelming his small staff, he had all but given up searching for the root cause of the epidemic and focused only on its effects. He continued to harbor a suspicion that squirrels in the East Bay had become a reservoir for infected fleas, but he had neither the time nor the men to act upon it.

All his attention was directed toward one number: 2 percent. Doctors treating an outbreak of plague in Manila had discovered that a roughly one-percent infection rate among the rat population resulted in approximately sixty human cases per month, a sizable but not overwhelming number. If the infection rate among rats rose above 2 percent, the disease exploded into the human population, leaving a trail of dead behind. Already, Blue had noted that 1.5 percent of the thousands of rats that passed through the Rattery each day were infected by plague, a rate that had tripled since his men had begun their collections three months earlier. As the infection rate edged closer and closer to its tipping point, Blue knew that he must start preparing to place the city under quarantine or risk watching plague consume the nation.

It was the last thing he wanted to do. Sealing off the city from the outside world so quickly after its tragedy would likely mean its death. When asked by one of his men whether quarantining the city would spur additional public support for the rat-killing program, Blue cut him off. "My friend, have you ever been in a quarantined city?" he asked. When the man replied that he had not, Blue responded, "Then you cannot realize what you are asking me to do. To place such a curse upon San Francisco would be worse than a hundred fires and earthquakes and I love this city too well to do her such a frightful hurt."

Time was working against him. The weather would grow warmer in just a few months, prompting rats to become bolder in their search for food and increase the likelihood of human contact. "Conditions are not improving as rapidly as I would like them to," Blue confessed in a telegram to Wyman. "There can be no doubt that the city is infected from one end to the other." If his men did not significantly reduce the numbers of rats before the spring, he warned, the city would be left staring at "an outbreak of unprecedented proportions."

CHAPTER 15

THE WORST CORNER OF HELL

Spring was four months away. As the weather grew warmer, fleas would start their breeding season and lay up to fifty eggs per day, creating millions more potential carriers of plague swarming through the city in search of a host. The thought kept Blue up at night. Every rat that survived past winter could not only undo all the work that his men had accomplished thus far, but end the lives of thousands more victims. "The work and the campaign have become so exacting that I scarcely have time to eat and sleep properly," Blue wrote to a colleague in Washington.

With his window of opportunity closing, Blue grasped for other ways to break the city out of its complacency. He asked Dr. George Evans, the president of the California State Medical Society, to organize a summit of the most prominent citizens in San Francisco, hoping that by speaking directly to those with power he could bypass the influence of the *Chronicle*. Evans sent out six hundred invitations; sixty people showed up. Blue, by now inured to the city's apathy in the face of danger, spoke in a dispassionate tone as he relayed how death was likely to spread in the coming months on a scale the city had never before seen. The rat remained the city's greatest threat and it would soon start multiplying, leaving no home, business or park safe when all it took was a bite from a nearly invisible flea to send a person to their grave, he said. He then presented a map showing the locations of victims of plague since the outbreak began in August, alongside the places where infected rats had been captured. The map was speckled from end to end, as if hit by a paintbrush dripping in red ink. Markers signifying a victim were found in every neighborhood, proving that skin color or social class offered no immunity.

The only sanitary part of the city was Chinatown, he told the men before him, and nothing would stop the disease unless the public changed its behavior to make the city less hospitable to rats and their fleas. The attendees, many of them physicians, passed a resolution calling on Mayor Taylor to appoint a committee that would galvanize public support for the rat eradication campaign. A second meeting, open to the general public, was planned for January 28, just ten days away. Blue held on to a faint hope that the common men and women of San Francisco would prove more willing to confront the disease when presented directly with the truth of the danger they were in, though he steeled himself for one more disappointment in a city that only seemed to offer them.

More than three hundred people squeezed into a ballroom in the Merchant Exchange Building, a fifteen-story granite Beaux-Arts skyscraper that had been completed two years before the earthquake and now, with its minimal damage and quick repairs, was widely considered a symbol of the city's rebirth. Spurred by the mayor's call for cooperation, nearly every commercial association in town had asked its members to attend, packing the room until it was close to overflowing. Blue, clad in his khaki dress uniform with a ceremonial gold sword hanging from his hip, watched from the side of the stage as the audience, already the largest he had ever addressed in his life, continued to grow. Reserved and amiable by default, his natural inclination was to blend in with a crowd, not to rustle it into action. Yet as he took the stage, he knew that this was his best and last chance to get the people of the city on his side.

He spoke in a soft monotone as he relayed the facts of the epidemic to the men and women sitting before him, many of whom
had never seen a truthful word of it mentioned in one of the city's
newspapers. More than seventy-five people, nearly all of them white,
had died from plague in a span of four months, proving that the disease knew no racial lines, he said. If the city did not kill enough rats,
there would be no telling how many more deaths were to come.
As it stood, 1.5 percent of all rats that his corps of men caught each
week were infected with plague. There was a strong chance that the
number would increase during the warmer months, edging the city
ever closer to the 2 percent tipping point, where there would be no
choice but to implement a citywide quarantine to protect the rest of
the country. The Health Department was already overwhelmed by
the demands of rebuilding the city; combatting the plague would
prove impossible if the residents of San Francisco did not play their
part. "Unless we obtain the support of the people, the task is hope-
less," Blue told his audience.

The room was silent. Not knowing whether he had made any
allies, Blue soldiered on, his voice, with its melodic Southern
drawl, never revealing the full extent of his desperation. He turned
his attention to the scheduled arrival in four months of the Great
White Fleet, an armada of sixteen steel steam-powered U.S. Navy
battleships—all painted white—that was then in the middle of a cir-
cumnavigation of the globe with fourteen thousand sailors aboard.
The fleet, intended by President Theodore Roosevelt to peaceably
demonstrate America's growing military and economic power to
the rest of the world, had departed Virginia in December and was
scheduled to arrive in San Francisco in May. The city expected that
the fleet's arrival through the Golden Gate would lead to newspaper
articles from one coast to the other spotlighting San Francisco's resurrection after the earthquake and fire, finally allowing it to put the
disaster behind it. The longest parade in the city's history was being
planned by former mayor James Phelan to mark the occasion, with
over three thousand soldiers and dozens of floats honoring pioneers

from the Gold Rush, while railroads and hotels announced that they expected record crowds.

"The first thing the admiral of the fleet will ask when he reaches this port will be 'What are the health conditions?' If it is not safe for the fleet to come into this port it may create trouble for us," Blue warned the men and women before him, carefully positioning himself on the city's side. Left unsaid was that if it was not safe for the fleet to land in San Francisco, it would continue up the coast for an extended stay in Seattle, raising the chances that the Navy would transfer its Pacific operations to that port. The threat sent a ripple through the audience. Governor James Gillett, whose election the year before with the help of the Southern Pacific led to rumors that he remained in the railroad's pockets, rose to address the crowd. "Now is the time for the people of this city to do what they can to avert the danger of a quarantine," he said. "The plague exists . . . we now have the plague at a point where we can control it. We must not wait until it controls us."

Whatever hesitancy remained in San Francisco to acknowledge the disease evaporated in the face of the national embarrassment of quarantine and the loss of the Great White Fleet. A lineup of the city's most prominent businesses, including Wells Fargo, the Southern Pacific Railroad, and Levi Strauss & Co., joined together in the following weeks to raise half a million dollars to privately finance a sanitation campaign to complement Blue's efforts. Soon an additional four hundred paid sanitary inspectors were roaming the streets, trapping and poisoning rats according to Blue's directives. The newly christened Citizen's Health Committee purchased more than $15,000 worth of rat traps and poison, in quantities so large that it bought cheese for use as bait in lots of three thousand pounds at a time. To further spur ordinary citizens to kill rats, it began offering bounties of twenty-five cents for every male and fifty cents for every female that was brought to one of its field offices, a ploy that turned gangs of boys across the city into amateur killing squads.

After years of battling the city's apathy, Blue finally had its trust.

"I started an agitation on plague to arouse the citizens to a sense of their danger," he wrote in a letter to his mother in February, unable to conceal his pride at discovering that he had within him the qualities of a leader. "This agitation has grown out of my control. The people are aroused. I am making six speeches a day. My staff is doing the same. I have received calls for addresses all over the state. I am about worn out but must keep the iron hot and the people demand that I must lead them."

Blue appeared in every meeting hall, business or pulpit that would have him, spreading the gospel of rat eradication. There must be a sudden famine of food available for rats, he told his audiences, which could largely be accomplished by simple actions such as keeping garbage cans covered. Only then would the animals, who were naturally clever enough to realize that they were unwanted, be desperate enough to take poison or venture out into the open. If you happened to come across a rat running in the street or near your office, it was your duty as a citizen to kill it, just as cowboys on the frontier considered it automatic to kill any coyote they encountered to protect their herds. The crowds grew larger, and Blue, tapping into a previously unknown eloquence, grew more passionate in his attempts to stir his listeners to action. In front of a crowd of more than a thousand freight handlers for the Southern Pacific, he thundered, "I intend to kill a rat or two myself tonight, and I want all of you to do the same. It is the noblest work you can do."

Aiming to cover more ground, Blue told his deputy, Colby Rucker, to speak to as many groups as he could. Rucker revealed a hidden gift as an animated public speaker, happily barnstorming through dozens of speeches a day. Blessed with a performer's gift for sizing up his audience, he tailored his speeches to focus on themes of humor or fear as the occasion warranted. In front of women's clubs, he relied on his innate charm, telling crowds with a broad grin, "When you look in your garbage pails, ladies, think of me!" At other times, he attempted to scare his audience into compliance, telling one gathering of businessmen that "This city is in danger of a quarantine and I want you to understand that if a quarantine is placed on San Francisco, you people will imagine yourself in the worst corner of hell. The days following the disaster of April 1906 will seem like a holiday picture compared to the days to be spent in a city quarantined for bubonic plague."

By March, Rucker's voice gave out, and he spent a week whispering from the stage. "Dr. Rucker has been simply invaluable," Blue wrote to his sister Kate. "I address audiences because I am compelled to; Rucker does it for the love of the thing. We call him 'garbage can Rucker' because that is his hobby."

Newspapers began running articles describing the best ways to keep a home rat-free, finally breaking through the wall of misinformation that Blue had been previously unable to scale. Within weeks, Blue noticed signs of progress. The streets were cleaner; the herds of rats that had until recently swarmed over the city's ruins had thinned. No new plague victims had been discovered, helping Blue keep the pressure from other states to institute a quarantine of San Francisco or all of California at bay.

Yet he knew that he must do more. Each day, he checked the infection rate among the hundreds of rats examined at the Rattery. Though it was not increasing, neither was it falling at the rate that he'd expected, making it impossible for him to silence the fear that all of his work would turn out to be nothing but show. He had already left San Francisco twice without fully eradicating the disease, and he could not face the idea of doing so again. Weekly newspaper reports on the progress of the Great White Fleet around the tip of South America and up the Pacific coast chased his thoughts, reminding him of a deadline that he could not miss.

He drew on what resources he had, including some that were newly acquired. The hours he spent talking with audiences and answering their questions about plague made San Francisco residents and officials more confident of his sincerity and more willing to help, elevating his social currency. Those bonds allowed him to do things that had remained out of reach for Kinyoun, who had rarely ventured beyond the confines of his Angel Island laboratory. Slowly, Blue shook San Francisco out of its habits, leaving a newer, more sanitary version in its place.

Change came in ways large and small. In the spring, Blue prodded the city health department to improve conditions at Butchertown, the name given to a den of slaughterhouses nestled next to the bay by Islais Creek, along the southeastern edge of the city. Hundreds of cattle each day were processed in low wooden buildings set on piers jutting over marshland, with the blood and remains of butchered animals falling between gaps in the floorboards to countless waiting rats below. Butchers considered the rodents a free scavenger service. Fat rats, some the size of small dogs, scurried beneath and through the slaughterhouses, in groups so large that they moved as if one squirming shadow. After inspectors flagged the problem, business owners invited reporters to watch as teams of men poured boiling water on dense herds of rats living under the slaughterhouses. The demonstration did nothing to convince the health board, and six slaughterhouses and several stables were condemned.

Soon, the rhythms of San Francisco subtly changed, as if it had fallen under the spell of a new conductor. Owners of backyard chicken coops were told to pour layers of concrete on their floors to keep out nesting rodents; fruit peddlers began receiving citations for tossing rotten wares into the street that had long been free meals for rats; yellow placards appeared on stores that failed sanitary inspections, warning customers to go elsewhere. In the Lobos Square refugee camp, hundreds of wooden shacks were rebuilt eighteen inches off the ground, allowing dogs and cats headroom beneath the floorboards to chase rats into their nests. The camp's rat problem soon ended, and no cases of plague were identified among its residents. In order to prevent the possibility that infected dead rats would cross the bay, the city temporarily banned all manure shipments out of San Francisco until every stable installed metal rat-proof bins.

Houses that stood over ground-floor stables were condemned and razed throughout the city, removing one of the few remaining

architectural relics of San Francisco's earliest days. Garbage collectors who were found to deposit loads anywhere other than the
crematory were punished by heavy fines, eliminating a persistent
source of chaos and filth. Women's clubs, meanwhile, prodded the
school board to set rat traps in the city's schools and disinfect every
building over the Easter break, and paid for inspectors to canvass San
Francisco's candy stores and penny arcades and warn children then
of the dangers of playing with rats. "It is the opinion of the sanitary
officials that no such undertaking could ever be as successful again
without the help this community received from its women," noted
Blue's later report on the cleanup effort.

By the middle of the spring, San Francisco seemed more vibrant,
as if the accumulated grime built up over its first half century had
been wiped away to reveal color for the first time. The mayor hosted
a feast for five hundred guests at tables set up in the middle of Front
Street between Washington and Jackson to celebrate the city's progress. Heaping bowls of gleaming tropical fruit adorned long tables
topped with white linens, their color chosen to underscore how little
dirt remained on the streets. "There was a time when we were not
awake to the need of vigilance in our civic life, but that has passed,
in its wake has come a mighty awakening that bids fair to make the
name of San Francisco renowned the world over," Mayor Taylor
told the gathering. Blue then gave a short address congratulating the
merchants in the district for their part in the sanitation campaign
before turning the crowd's attention to Rucker. The women of the
neighborhood "deserve all the credit, because they have made the
men work," he began, to a mixture of laughter and applause.

There had not been a human victim of plague discovered in
months, yet Blue could not let himself relax even as he walked
through a city that was the cleanest it had ever been. Scores of
infected rats passed through his headquarters each day, meaning that
whatever progress he had made could turn out to be nothing but a
temporary lull. "I fear an outbreak by the advent of dry weather,"
he wrote in a letter to his sister Kate that March. He knew that the

city's support could be fickle and if he did not eliminate the disease soon he might not have another chance. Failure, he wrote, would doom San Francisco to "have a plague scare every summer for the next twenty years."

He was willing to try anything. Intent on proving his suspicions that rodents were migrating from one neighborhood to another, Blue gathered dozens of plague-free rats and dyed their fur. Crimson rats were released into one half of the city, while green rats were let go in another. His men then posted flyers around the city, urging citizens to report any sightings of brightly colored rodents. Blue knew that there was a warren of sewer lines and unused water pipes running under the city; perhaps, this ploy might enable him to gather enough information to sketch out their shape and pinpoint where to lay more traps.

In his desperation to track rats, Blue gave no thought to the press reaction. He was blindsided when the *Chronicle* gleefully mocked the program, eroding some of the goodwill he had built up over the last few weeks of success. "If you should see a tiny mouse, whose hide was salmon pink, would you not join the temperance band, and blame it on the drink? Fear not these harmless little things that scurry round and squeal; they're all in Dr. Blue's employ, and all of them are real," the paper wrote in a front-page verse. Thanks to Blue's efforts, "the rainbow rat will probably be the rat of the future, or some weird progeny will result from the union of rats of different colors," it added.

Blue quietly shut down the experiment before gleaning anything of value from it. Yet his problems with the press were only beginning. In late April, Dr. Halstead Stansfield, who had until recently been Blue's chief bacteriologist, walked into the fog-shrouded forest of eucalyptus trees on Mount Sutro, a nine-hundred-foot hill in the heart of the city, with a revolver in his pocket. Stansfield had resigned his post after the death of his wife and young son sent him into a deep depression, and in his months off of the force had sought comfort in alcohol, which only sent him spiraling further into despair. In a small clearing off of the main path, Stansfield shot himself in the head. His body was discovered two days later by two men out for an afternoon walk.

Those who had been frustrated in their efforts to undermine Blue and the changes he was implementing pounced upon Stansfield's death, seeking to cast his suicide as evidence that federal health officers were not to be trusted. "The evidence was indisputable that Dr. Stansfield had been erratic for a long time and his melancholia was intensified by intemperance. Yet it is upon the scientific findings of this mentally unhinged specialist that Dr. Blue and his associate plague experts pronounced San Francisco as suffering from an epidemic," wrote the *Wasp*, a weekly political magazine known for its hatred of the Chinese. The *Chronicle*, meanwhile, argued in the week following Stansfield's death that the rat eradication campaign was meaningless. In an editorial likely demanded by de Young, it asserted that "There is no reason to believe that the health of this city will be materially affected one way or another by the slaughter of rats, for which the money is being extorted from us by the threat of quarantining the city . . . The doctors accuse the rats because they cannot find any other means of dissemination."

In response, Blue issued a report showing that not only had there not been a case of bubonic plague discovered in the last ninety days, but that overall death rates in the city were declining. The paper then changed its approach, insisting instead that the city was too clean, and ran a series of articles mocking what it called "the sanitarians."

Blue ignored the provocation, focusing instead on the imminent arrival of the Great White Fleet. Over the previous three weeks, the infection rate among rats examined at the Rattery had fallen to 1.2 percent. Although encouraging, that number proved that the danger had not yet passed. There were still thousands of infected rats running beneath the city's streets, and all it would take was for one flea to jump onto a human's skin for the panic to begin anew.

Everything in his training told Blue to keep the port closed rather than risk the infection spreading aboard a contingent of battleships that had become a symbol of the nation's power. Yet as he looked across the city, he saw in its rebirth hope for his own life. San Francisco had buoyed him when his marriage to Juliette crumbled and given him a new sense of purpose. Though he would not admit it to others in the Service, he had begun to consider the possibility of living in the city permanently after the plague campaign was over.

Without consulting Wyman, Blue issued a clean bill of health for the port that allowed the festivities to go on as planned, and prayed that he would not regret it.

CHAPTER 16

ONE OF CALIFORNIA'S
ADOPTED SONS

The wave of visitors streaming toward San Francisco was so great that railroads had to add special trains from Oregon, Utah, Nevada and Washington to meet the demand, each one packed with passengers intent on seeing with their own eyes what was being called the most powerful naval force ever assembled in the Pacific. In the week before its arrival, the number of daily riders on ferries crossing San Francisco Bay jumped by nearly half a million, assembling the raw material for what would later be called the largest gathering in the city's history. On May 6, 1908, an estimated crowd of one million people crammed onto the hills of San Francisco, jostling and jumbling like ants as they tried to secure a view of the bay. As if answering a thousand unspoken prayers, the morning fog relented and burned away, leaving nothing but the shimmering dark water and the wide blue sky.

The first ships came into view through the Golden Gate shortly before noon. From a distance, they looked like moving firestacks shooting dark plumes of smoke into the sky. As the boats came closer, the massive guns of the city's seaside forts roared in salute. Soon, a six-mile-long parade of blinding white warships stretched from the Golden Gate past the island of Alcatraz and looped back away from the city's waterfront toward the open Pacific. Vessels from the Pacific Fleet joined in the procession, increasing the size of the armada to forty-six vessels. Spectators gave up trying to take them all in, overwhelmed by a collection that included more than a dozen battleships, several armored cruisers, three torpedo boats and a single hospital ship.

Before the fleet had left Virginia at the start of its round-the-world voyage, its commander, Rear Admiral Robley D. Evans, had told reporters, "We are ready at the drop of a hat for a feast, a frolic or a fight." San Francisco, of all places, knew how to provide all three. A miles-long parade ran down Mission Street to mark the occasion, followed by a ball at the Fairmont Hotel that went on for two days. Each of the fifteen thousand sailors who disembarked were handed a cigar as soon as he stepped on shore, along with a pamphlet listing all of the city's attractions. Not included among them were the bars and brothels of the former Barbary Coast, though most sailors needed no instructions on how to get there.

Those who sought tamer escapes headed toward the three-story Naval Club House, built by volunteers in the weeks ahead of the fleet's arrival on an open lot two blocks from the waterfront. Rooms on the first two floors were stuffed with entertainments ranging from pool tables to free writing paper, yet its third floor was the main draw: 250 clean cots, with fresh pillows and sheets, where a sailor could stay the night for the price of twenty-five cents. Volunteers organized free tours of the city and Golden Gate Park in opentop convertibles, giving some sailors their first experience of riding in the still-novel invention of an automobile. Trains decorated with flowers from end to end ferried others on day trips to Stanford University, San José and Vallejo, where booming brass bands greeted them at every stop.

Never one for military pageantry, Blue kept a low profile during the fleet's three-week-long stay in San Francisco. He remained huddled in the Fillmore Street laboratory, where he kept watch on the daily tallies of infected rats collected by his staff. Every night he went to sleep fearing a call that a sailor from the fleet had become infected with plague; every morning he told himself that he had only received an additional day's reprieve and nothing more, starting the cycle of worry over anew. His fortieth birthday came and went without notice. He extracted himself from his lab rotation only to serve as best man at the wedding of his friend Captain Edmund Shortlidge, an assistant surgeon at an Army base in the city. Once the ceremony was over, he returned in his full dress uniform to his lab, not wanting to waste any more time.

It wasn't until the Great White Fleet set sail for Seattle that Blue allowed himself to relax. No plague victims were discovered during the fleet's stay or on any of its ships in the weeks following departure, leaving San Francisco's celebration of its revival unblemished. He was once again free to concentrate on eradicating the disease without the fear that he had been complicit in spreading it to sailors who were bound for other ports around the world, accelerating the epidemic. His mind clear, he turned his focus from rats to their fleas, searching for a clue that would help him understand more about how the plague bacilli spread. He ordered his ratcatchers to bring back as many living rodents as they could. In the laboratory the writhing animals were doused in chloroform, killing them and any parasites still clinging to their bodies. Doctors then combed through their fur, extracting fleas. The insects were placed in glass jars and labeled with the date and district where they were captured.

A researcher on Blue's staff by the name of Carroll Fox collected thousands of specimens and began examining each one under the microscope. He soon realized that the most common flea in the city was the Northern European species, *Ceratophyllus fasciatus*, rather than *Pulex cheposis*, which was the most prevalent in plague-infested ports such as Hong Kong and Bombay. The discovery suggested that most of the fleas in the city had arrived either overland or aboard ships from the Atlantic, rather than from rats hiding on ships from Hawaii and Asia.

Their point of origin was only one part of the Fox's discovery.

The main difference between the two species is in the layout of their guts: the Indian rat flea has a spiny ridge in its abdomen where blood from its most recent meal collects, eventually blocking material from reaching the stomach. That clot leads the famished insect to aggressively bite any living mammal that it encounters. Fresh blood helps to dislodge the clot, spurring the flea to essentially vomit some of the material stalled in its belly into the skin of its new victim. The host inevitably scratches the site of the bite, pushing the blood from the flea's previous meals deeper into his or her own bloodstream.

A *Pulex cheposis* that feeds on a plague-infected victim retains the bacilli of the disease in the blood clot in its gut. Each bite thereafter brings new blood into its digestive tract and ejects some of the plague-infected material into the body of a new victim, introducing *Yersinia pestis* into another bloodstream where it can multiply and eventually take over. The European flea, by comparison, retains less blood in its stomach, leaving it less likely to develop a blockage that prompts it to attack as aggressively. When it does bite, the flea deposits only a fraction of its stomach material into the body of its new host, minimizing its ability to spread infection compared with its more ravenous Asian cousin.

Though Blue and his men did not realize it, they had finally answered the question of why the disease did not spread in San Francisco as rapidly as it had in Asia. Thanks to the gut structure of its most common flea, the carriers of the disease were biting less aggressively and when they did attack they did not inject as much of the plague bacilli into their new hosts. Only the year before, a study published in the *Calcutta Journal of Medicine* had hinted at the increased role that *Pulex cheposis* played in the spread of the disease compared with other varieties of the insect. "There is much in favour of *Pulex cheposis* playing an active part in the transfer of plague from the rat to man . . . There can be no doubt that *Pulex cheposis*, unlike *Pulex fasciatus*, another common rat flea, bites man."

San Francisco had unwittingly served as a seven-year experiment, showing what would happen if the pandemic devouring Hong Kong and India came to a port where a different species of flea was more prevalent. The slow spread of the disease—a phenomenon that led the city to doubt Kinyoun's warnings and call the epidemic a fake ploy by corrupt health officials—had hinged on the stomach of a flea, a lucky quirk that spared an untold number of lives.

In July, Blue celebrated the six-month mark since the discovery of the last human victim of the plague. There had been no outbreak in the spring and early summer as he had feared and—barring any sudden resurgence—he could see that his mission would soon be winding down. For the first time since his emergency posting to San Francisco the previous September, he realized that there were other aspects of life that he might be missing. "My work may be satisfactorily completed by late fall, and I may then return to the 'Effete East' in quest of other adventures," he wrote to his sister Kate. "On the other hand, the disease may reappear and hold me in the 'Golden West' for six months longer . . . Tell Mother that I am still single but that the 'fair heads' out here are very hard to resist."

Thousands of rats were still examined at the Rattery each week, and the rate of infection continued to fall. By the end of summer, it was common to go a week or two without observing a single diseased rat among the more than five thousand corpses spliced open each day by federal doctors in the Fillmore Street laboratory. In October, what proved to be the last infected rat in San Francisco was discovered in a fruit warehouse. After several more weeks of plague-free rat specimens confirmed it, the disease seemed to be finally eradicated from the city. Blue and Wyman officially declared San Francisco a healthy port that November, leading the *Call* to blare in a front-page headline, "Clean Bill of Health Given San Francisco; Surgeon General Wyman Reports Pacific Coast States Free from Plague."

As Blue looked out over the city, there were few parts of San Francisco's daily life in which he could not see his reflection. More than 250,000 square feet of wooden boardwalks had been replaced with rat-proof concrete sidewalks at his insistence; over six million square feet of buildings in the city were now supported by concrete floors; more than 11,000 houses had been disinfected and their backyards cleared of any material that could provide shelter to rodents. Just as important was what a visitor to San Francisco could no longer see: Blue's rat eradication campaign had killed more than two million rats, a number five times the size of the city's human population. More than 154,000 of those rats had passed across the long metal dissection tables of the Rattery. The city, once notorious for its filth and frontier mindset, was now one of the most modern and sanitary metropolises in the world.

After so many years of struggle, Blue finally had a reason to celebrate. On March 31, 1909, four hundred men clad in tuxedos gathered in a grand banquet hall at the Fairmont Hotel for a dinner held in his honor. Women in formal gowns clustered at tables along the balcony railing, overlooking the floor below. Blue took his place at a long table at the front of the room, with Governor Gillett on one side of him and Mayor Taylor on the other. Homer King, the president of the Bank of California and the head of the Citizens Health Committee, presided as the evening's master of ceremonies. Reporters from every newspaper in the city were on hand, as well as representatives from several Eastern publications whose respect San Francisco still longed for. A copy of the 313-page report partly written by Blue and Rucker that described how San Francisco had conquered plague was placed at every setting, bound in a brilliant red cover. "The people of San Francisco have the satisfaction of knowing that they protected not merely their city, but the whole country at large," it began. "Had anti-plague measures failed here the spread of the disease would have been extremely difficult to control. Therefore, the cities and states of the union should, and we believe do, join with us in gratification at the happy outcome."

The banquet proceeded through several courses, each one touching on one part of Blue's cleanup campaign. The oysters were not blue points, the menu noted, because "He's been giving them to us for two years." The vegetables were "fresh from our produce district. We spread out tables in the street down there and call it 'Spotless Town.'" Ice cream was served in the shape of a mousetrap with the head of a fake rat protruding below it, while drinks came in glasses the shape of miniature garbage cans.

Speakers lined up to toast Blue and the work of his men, highlighting how Blue had brought about change through tact and amiability, rather than through force of personality. He led the city by showing a willingness to speak directly to its citizens, rather than by insisting upon directives from an isolated laboratory on Angel Island, and the city returned the respect. "You are here to learn what Dr. Rupert Blue has done for your city; how his leadership asserted itself at the time when a leader was most needed," King said. More praise followed, leaving Blue, a man unaccustomed to public spectacles, embarrassed by the attention. "We made no mistake when we chose him to clean up our city," said Governor Gillett. "It is now up to you, citizens of San Francisco, never to let disease again enter your city." Then Walter Macarthur, who would soon take on the position of U.S. Shipping Commissioner, rose to his feet and said, "We owe the success of our sanitation campaign to the fact that Dr. Blue carried no 'big stick.' Dr. Blue manifested in that campaign the very highest qualities of leadership. As soon as he realized that the people of San Francisco were disposed to pay heed to the rules as laid down he found his course easy."

As Blue finally approached the lectern, a cheer arose and continued for a full five minutes, only dying down once King implored the crowd to let the man speak. When calm was finally restored, Blue thanked the city for putting its trust in him. "I feel as if I were one of California's adopted sons," he began. "Need I say that I am profoundly grateful for this evidence of your appreciation? Need I say that the campaign would not have been successful had it not been for the cooperation of your citizens? . . . San Francisco has fought her battle and as one of you I am proud of the victory she has gained."

When Blue finished speaking, Mayor Taylor presented him with a gold watch, an inscription on the back thanking him for his service to the city. Every member of Blue's staff was given a medal, which the mayor pinned to their chests in front of the cheering crowd. Other banquets followed in the weeks ahead, with Blue and his men toasted in so many elegant restaurants, churches and meeting rooms that they began to lose count, happily allowing the feeling of victory to wash over them after so many lonely hours of worry.

For all the celebrations, Blue knew that the victory over plague was partial at best. Though the disease was no longer present in the city, it still remained lurking in the hills of the East Bay. In August of 1907, a seven-year-old boy named Joe Farias had died of what appeared to be plague on the family's ranch near the town of Concord in Contra Costa County. Two more victims were discovered in the same area within the same week. Federal health agents learned from local ranchers that thick herds of sickly squirrels were appearing on farms throughout the county, moving so slowly that all it took to kill them was a stick.

Blue, at the time still focused on the danger facing San Francisco, had sent Rucker to investigate. He discovered a dead rat on a ranch a mile and a half from the home of the first victim and brought its body back to the Fillmore Street headquarters. Tests confirmed that it had died of the disease.

Rucker began making more forays into the East Bay, each time bringing additional men with him to fan out across the golden hills. It was on one of these expeditions that federal health officers came upon a wild ground squirrel, still alive, that appeared to be suffering from the disease. A tissue sample taken from its body proved that the animal was infected with plague. Researchers had long known that fleas in laboratories could spread the disease from rats to squirrels, yet it had never before been observed in the wild. Now, with proof before him, Blue realized that the perimeter of the outbreak had widened. "The discovery has caused considerable apprehension," he wrote to Wyman in Washington.

The danger was twofold. Ground squirrels were abundant throughout the state, creating a deep reservoir of victims that the disease could infect. Capturing and killing them in large quantities was made close to impossible not only by their physical abilities—a squirrel can run at over 12 miles per hour, roughly double the speed of an average adult human, and jump over ten horizontal feet, making it small and quick enough to dodge a bullet—but by the fact that their colonies are often spread across a warren of underground tunnels more than thirty feet in length, neutralizing the effectiveness of poison. Squirrels that could be caught were widely consumed as food by rural families, putting humans in direct contact with flea-infested fur. In some rural parts of the state, impoverished families had no other source of meat.

Blue only had to look across the bay to the foothills of the East Bay framing the horizon to be reminded that plague was still out there, searching for its next victim. He gave his men a week to enjoy their success in eradicating it from San Francisco. Then he announced that Rucker would be in charge of chasing the disease before it spread deeper into the continent.

Just as Blue had done in his rat eradication campaign in San Francisco, Rucker improvised, searching for anything that could help him replicate their success in the city. He began experimenting with the best type and composition of poison gas to fumigate the animals' burrows. When poison proved ineffective, he turned to explosives, hoping to blast the danger away. While the use of dynamite did help, the sound and vibrations often scared the squirrels that survived into fleeing, dispersing the disease even more. Only after discovering that squirrels can withstand a higher dose of strychnine in their cheeks than their stomachs did he begin to make headway. He placed traps of poisoned barley far away from squirrels' nests, allowing the chemical to saturate the animal's mouth while it carried the tainted food back to others in its nest, where it would become lethal once it was swallowed.

Rucker knew that what federal health officials had learned in combating plague in the dense urban environment of San Francisco would likely offer little or no help when facing acres of wild, untouched land. "It is in these regions that the hardest part of the fighting must occur," Rucker wrote. "Such a campaign will be an enormous undertaking, but it must come, and not until it has reached a successful close can we hope for the answer to the piteous prayer which has gone up from mankind since the dawn of life—that no plague may come nigh our dwelling."

CHAPTER 17

CAST ASIDE

For the first time since he was a child, Blue felt at home.
With the city no longer mired in an epidemic, he closed the makeshift laboratory and Rattery at Fillmore Street and opened a new headquarters in a rebuilt downtown skyscraper on New Montgomery. There, the miracle of San Francisco's rebirth was impossible to ignore. Where two years before lay only rubble was now a thriving, modern commercial district, the economic heart of one of the most important cities on the Pacific. After years of working in cramped, unheated rooms while piloting the city's revival, Blue treated himself to a wide wooden desk and a broad oriental rug from W. & J. Sloane, an upscale New York furniture dealer that counted John D. Rockefeller among its clients. The campaign to eradicate plague from the state's ground squirrel population would take months, if not years, he reasoned, anchoring him in the city for the foreseeable future.

With Rucker at his side, he spent weeks driving across the broad farms and rolling hills of Northern California, tracking the eastward spread of the disease. Despite the acres of open land, its path was easy to trace. Ranchers would first notice that something was wrong when dozens of emaciated squirrels would emerge from a burrow and stagger about as if in a daze. The fur of the diseased animals would appear to have been brushed back against the grain, while their jaws looked swollen and dislodged. They would then die off in such great numbers that their holes would become jammed with dead bodies, with carcasses lying in heaps around the blocked entrance. Flocks of buzzards feasted upon the remains, widening the spectacle. Those not consumed by birds were eaten by coyotes and rattlesnakes, leaving nothing behind.

By the middle of 1909, infected squirrels could be found across 1,500 square miles of the state, an area more than thirty times larger than San Francisco. The only thing preventing a human epidemic in the region was its emptiness: four times as many people lived in San Francisco itself as in the quilt of counties stretching from Contra Costa south and eastward to the Nevada state line, with mountainous Alpine County serving as home to just 309 people. Sixteen patients developed plague in the region in the year following the disease's retreat from San Francisco, eight of them dying from the disease. The methods that had saved the city—covering and removing trash quickly to cut back on the food supply, ample use of poison, and rebuilding cellars and chicken coops with concrete—would have no effect in a region made up mostly of farms and acres of untouched land.

Once again, Blue had to innovate. In order to reduce the amount of human contact with potential carriers of the disease, he convinced the state health board to ban the shipment of ground squirrels within California unless they were for scientific purposes, eliminating the widespread market for the animals as food. An inspector was stationed at the entrance to the tunnel connecting Oakland with Contra Costa County to warn trappers ferrying bags of dead squirrels to sell as meat of the danger they were exposing themselves to by handling the animals. Blue then rehired dozens of his former ratcatchers. He gave each one a rifle and a canvas knapsack and told them to spend a week in the East Bay and send back as many dead squirrels as they could. One man killed 131 squirrels in eight hours, each of which was tagged with the location where it was shot and sealed in a tin can pumped with chloroform to kill its fleas. Crates full of tin cans containing dead squirrels began arriving at the San Francisco office each afternoon, along with an occasional milk jug stuffed with bodies when trappers ran out of supplies and improvised.

Federal doctors once again began the bloody work of slicing open the chest of each animal and searching its organs for signs of plague. By August of 1909, 178 infected squirrels had passed through the laboratory, leaving Blue to estimate that 1.2 percent of the squirrel population of the East Bay carried the disease. Though still below the 2 percent rate signaling that a human epidemic was near, it only confirmed his fears. All it would take was for the fleas of an infected squirrel to jump on to a passing hiker or a family dog for the disease to travel to Oakland or Berkeley, once again introducing plague into an urban environment where it could easily find new victims.

Blue launched a statewide campaign to create what he called "squirrel-free zones" around California's major cities, hoping to stave off another outbreak by reducing the number of wild squirrels—estimated at 100 million—living in the state. Landowners in the roughly mile-wide barriers were urged to dynamite all squirrel holes on their property, while health officials spread poison liberally, covering more than one thousand acres of Contra Costa County with tainted grain. Blue trained corps of trappers—many of them men who had seen military service in the Spanish American War and felt comfortable with a gun—in the habits and preferences of squirrels and urged them to kill as many as possible. "As the conditions stand today, it is evident that nothing short of a relentless campaign of rodent extermination can prevent the epizootic from spreading over the entire State," Blue said in an address to the powerful Fruit Growers Convention in Stockton. "As long as there is one case in a country the whole world is afraid of it."

Still the disease spread outward. Trappers in San Joaquin, Stanislaus, and Merced counties found infected squirrels, as if it was traveling along vines emanating out of San Francisco and down the state. An infected squirrel was then found in the central California coastal county of San Luis Obispo, often considered the unofficial dividing line between the more populated northern and faster-growing southern halves of the state. Concerned that an urban outbreak would be next, Blue sent trappers into Los Angeles, Riverside, Orange and San Bernardino counties to assess the risk. The bodies of more than twelve thousand squirrels were shipped back to his laboratory. No evidence of plague was found, though Blue worried that it was only a matter of time.

Though his fears were rising, Blue had to concede more control of the squirrel campaign to his deputies. Now known as the savior of San Francisco, Blue was increasingly called away from his post whenever the Marine Hospital Service encountered a fearsome epidemic around the globe. He sailed down to the Chilean coastal town of Iquique when an outbreak of plague claimed more than a hundred victims, and spent weeks in Panama battling an outbreak of yellow fever. In each, he instituted sanitation methods similar to those that had worked in San Francisco. His reputation and personality served as a halo around the Service's efforts, buffering local objections to the presence of federal health officers.

Blue was attempting to control a wave of yellow fever in Hawaii when, in November of 1911, he received word from Rucker that Wyman was dead. The failing health of the Surgeon General had long been an open secret within the Service, though no one dared to comment publicly on the future of a man who considered any remark on his status nothing less than betrayal. Overweight and diabetic, Wyman had increasingly cloistered himself in his office, rarely attending Service functions or meeting with officers in the field. Yet it was the sapping of his ambition that truly signaled that his life was nearing its end. Where he had once rushed to claim any additional federal mandate in hopes of making the Service into a more important agency, Wyman had in recent months dismissed new opportunities without regret, rejecting a proposal to create a

Children's Bureau within the Service that would provide care for new mothers and their infants by calling it merely sentimental.

Unwilling to the end to cede power, Wyman did not nominate a successor, upending the forty-year tradition of the office in which the outgoing Surgeon General chose his replacement. His death left the Service in a panic. Knowing that Blue would be too reticent to lobby for the job himself, Rucker sent Blue a telegram stating simply, "Wyman dead. Have entered you in race. Too late [to] back out now." Blue replied quickly, "Go to it."

Though he was the most famous officer in the Service, Blue was not the unanimous choice to lead it. Several high-ranking officials lobbied instead for Joseph White, the senior officer to whom Wyman had first turned when he removed Joseph Kinyoun from San Francisco, to take the helm. Each man had his supporters: White was seen as the better pure doctor; Blue, the more collegial. President William Howard Taft, then in his second year in office, was left to make the decision, and joked with reporters that he would have to pick his favorite color.

In the end he was swayed by Blue's record of twice eliminating plague from San Francisco, a job that White had called impossible. Blue was told to return from Hawaii and make his way to Washington, where he met with the president at the White House. Shortly thereafter, Taft announced that at the age of forty-six Blue would become the nation's fourth Surgeon General, heading an agency whose name would now be simply the U.S. Public Health Service.

The scope of the job was staggering. Blue, who had never overseen more than a dozen officers at any one time, stepped into the top seat of a bureaucracy encompassing a staff of more than a thousand, ranging from pharmacists to nurses to engineers. Simply listing his responsibilities required a map of the world. He was in charge of 50 quarantine stations along the U.S. coasts, 120 medical relief stations spread from Japan to Africa, a leprosy treatment center in Hawaii and a tuberculosis sanitarium in New Mexico. The geography of the job was one thing; its new sense of purpose another. As part of the restructuring that included the name change, the Service's mission had been expanded to include not just infectious diseases like cholera and plague but "all diseases of man," a nod toward the optimism that pervaded medicine at the time. Sanitation, bacteriology and the development of the first modern drugs had made it seem possible that life would one day be if not eternal then something close to it. Blue's agency was expected not only to prevent epidemics of virulent disease from surfacing in America but to attend to anything that could improve the nation's quality of life.

In his first years in the job, Blue directed investigations into pollution in drinking water, oversaw an expansion of worker safety laws, pushed for more stringent milk pasteurization codes and blocked the sale of so-called "cure-alls" by charlatans who claimed that their secret mixtures could succeed where other medicines had failed. To strengthen the trust between patients and doctors, he lobbied the American Medical Association to adopt a new code of ethics which stated in part that "it is unprofessional to promise radical cures; to boast of cures of secret methods of treatment or remedies," a creed credited with professionalizing the ranks of doctors. He fought typhoid fever in Iowa and Virginia, smallpox in Kentucky and dengue fever in Florida, and organized the first meeting held in the United States of the International Congress on Hygiene and Demography, which brought thirty-three nations to Washington to share their successes in what was then being called the Sanitary Movement.

The gathering, the largest of its kind, showed the first glimpses of a future in which human life was expected to be long and meaningful. The attendees were nearly all born in the harsher world of the nineteenth century, when rudimentary care and poor sanitation led many parents to bury their children before they reached adolescence. Educators demonstrated the benefits of schools with more natural light; hospitals gave seminars on how teaching mothers to care for their infants improved mortality rates; sanitariums built scale models showcasing the use of calming colors and bubbling fountains in rooms dedicated to the treatment of the mentally ill, a break from the metal cages that some psychotic patients were locked inside just a generation before. In addition to leading the conference, Blue spoke to packed audiences about how his rat eradication campaign had not only eliminated plague from San Francisco but cut down on the spread of illness overall.

He made time for more pedestrian health matters, too, by installing drinking fountains in government buildings in Washington to prevent the use of shared cups that easily spread disease. Concerned about the growing prevalence among poor Southerners of pellagra—a painful skin disease that progresses from diarrhea to skin lesions to dementia and death—he established the Spartanburg Pellagra Hospital in South Carolina, the nation's first clinic devoted to studying the effects of the disease. He asked Dr. Joseph Goldberger, then known as one of the Service's best officers in the field of infectious disease, to search for its root cause.

At the time, most doctors considered the disease the result of a parasite, though it had never been identified. Goldberger, however, was struck by the fact that doctors and nurses who treated pellagra patients never fell ill themselves. Its victims were overwhelmingly concentrated among poor sharecroppers and African Americans who ate filling but nutrient-poor diets consisting mostly of corn. Sensing that the cause was nutrient deficiency, Goldberger ran experiments at orphanages in which he discovered that giving children milk and eggs in addition to their standard meals resulted in fewer cases. Other tests soon revealed that adult patients with the disease who were given more balanced diets including turkey, chicken and green peas almost universally recovered. When skeptics argued that diet alone could not prevent the disease, Goldberger injected himself with blood and other bodily fluids from patients, proving that it was not transmissible. Though he would not live to see it, later experiments proved that the disease was caused by a lack of niacin, a common B vitamin.

Uninterested as he was in power or glory, Blue was the opposite of what the Service had long expected from its Surgeon Generals. Gamesmanship and political maneuvering remained foreign to him, and he exhibited a humility and earnestness that often felt out of place in Washington. Where Wyman had valued control, Blue knew that his talent lay not in his scientific certainty but in his willingness to listen to others, and was content to let others take the reins where warranted. The effect was an immediate boost in the agency's morale, leaving one doctor to credit Blue with fostering "the spirit that makes every man on the corps go where he is ordered on a minute's notice and put in twenty-four hours a day instead of the regulation seven whenever there is the slightest public reason for it." His reputation grew so high that he was nominated president of the American Medical Association, the first time that the Surgeon General had also headed the largest organization of private physicians in the country.

The demands of Blue's dizzying schedule began to manifest themselves in his body, turning the boxer's build that he had long prided himself on into the wide frame more common among men of his stature who were approaching the age of fifty. He lamented the amount of time he spent shuffling between meetings in Washington, a life so different from the solitary, peripatetic lifestyle that had become second nature to him. "All seasons and days are alike to me," he complained in a letter to his sister Sallie.

When given an opportunity to rejoin the front lines he took it. On July 28, 1914—the day that Austria–Hungary declared war on Serbia, effectively starting the First World War—a forty-nine-year-old Swedish sailor by the name of Charles Lundene died in an isolation ward at Charity Hospital in New Orleans after developing a high fever and dark, swollen glands on his groin. An autopsy confirmed doctors' suspicions: the body was bristling with plague, making Lundene the first known person in the eastern half of the country to die from the disease. A second victim was discovered the next day, prompting the mayor to request help from Washington to quash what looked like the beginning of an epidemic.

Blue ordered Rucker and a team of men who had worked with him in San Francisco to report to the city and boarded a train himself, arriving in the city two days later. There was little time to waste. New Orleans was the gateway for all traffic up and down the Mississippi, connecting the farms and factories of the Midwest with ports around the world. Infected fleas that jumped onto a rat hiding on a ship heading northward could spread the disease to Memphis, St. Louis and St. Paul within a week. If the outbreak was not contained quickly and it was necessary to impose a quarantine, then the country's chief connection to the Panama Canal—scheduled to open in less than a month—would be shuttered, denting its economy at a time of war.

In the first hours of the outbreak, Charity Hospital was evacuated and its patients sent into quarantine at a former plantation north of the city. Health officials then dragged all of the furniture outside and burned it in a bonfire on St. Joseph Street. Patients who were suspected of developing plague were isolated and injected with a newly developed anti-plague serum that seemed to shock the disease out of the body, leaving one man who received an injection after his fever spiked to 108 degrees soon shivering with a 96-degree chill that required nurses to replace ice packs around his body with hot water bottles.

Once Blue arrived, he set up a laboratory next to City Hall and followed the same script which had helped save San Francisco. He dispatched more than 350 ratcatchers across the city, while paying special attention to the Stuyvesant Docks off of Tchoupitoulas Street, where shipments of grain from the Midwest attracted thousands of rats. Every rodent that was caught was brought back to Blue's laboratory, where it was tagged with the location and date of its capture and autopsied. Blue went through the city, identifying all of the ways in which it harbored the animals. Outhouses and backyard chicken coops were torn down; homes were raised off of the ground; layers of concrete were laid underneath sidewalks and buildings.

Blue spent two months in New Orleans, enough time to ensure

that there was no widespread outbreak. He then traveled to New York, Philadelphia and other major cities along the East Coast, implementing rat-proofing measures in hopes of preventing plague from nestling into the densest urban centers of the country. In Philadelphia, public health officials offered bounties of five cents for every live rat—and two cents for a dead one—brought to a receiving station at the Race Street pier and posted handbills around the city urging residents to "Kill The Rats—And Prevent the Plague." "Every one of our seaports is now menaced by this frightful disease," Blue told the *New York Times*.

He continued to direct New Orleans's rat control campaign from Washington. After discovering that the Egyptian rat, a species known for its climbing ability, was more common in the city than the Norway rat he had encountered in San Francisco, he ordered homes and businesses to insert a layer of metal in their roofs, preventing rodents from eating through the ceiling in search of food. He had signs hung up around the city depicting cartoon rats in top hats and tuxedos feasting out of an uncovered trash bin underneath foot-high letters asking, "Is Your House Rat Proof?" In the eighteen months that Public Health Service officials were in New Orleans, they killed and autopsied nearly 375,000 rats, a sum almost equal to the total human population of the city. Approximately thirty people developed plague, ten of them fatally.

Though his work to combat plague kept him consumed with what he considered a disease of the past, Blue continued to look toward the future. The new era of medicine that the Public Health Service was helping usher in was taking medical care out of the home and the offices of country doctors and centering it on the hospital, an institution that until the end of the nineteenth century was considered the last resort for those who had no means or family to support them. Procedures that would have seemed nothing short of fantasy a generation before were performed daily in urban operating rooms, drawing on sophisticated technology that felt otherworldly to patients whose parents had largely lived by candlelight.

The danger in such a rush of invention was that not all Americans would benefit. Blue, unable to forget his sisters in Marion to whom he continued to send monthly checks, began advocating for a national system of health insurance to bring the wonders of the modern era within the reach of poor farmers and factory workers who were the most likely to be exposed to illness. "There are unmistakable signs that health insurance will constitute the next great step in social legislation," he told a meeting of the American Medical Association in Detroit in June of 1916 to great applause.

Along with legislation, he brought modern medicine and science to areas that had been left behind. In order to let skeptical Americans see it for themselves, he funded a special train that traveled to rural outposts and set up demonstrations of the positive effects of sanitation. One train car displayed models of hygienic toilets; in another, early motion pictures showed how to exterminate rats, mosquitoes and other common carriers of disease. The work served as a useful distraction from the reports detailing the effects of chemical weapons on soldiers in Europe that filtered onto his desk in Washington. "I never thought that I would live to see such a colossal war that is prevailing in Europe," he wrote in a letter back home. "It is simply barbarous."

The U.S. entry into the war in 1917 changed the course of Blue's life. As the first American soldiers prepared to ship out for the battlefields of Europe, Congress debated whether to fold the Public Health Service into the military. Blue offered no strong opinion on the Service's future, planting seeds of distrust among officers who were put off by what they considered his apathy. The Service eventually remained independent, but further demands from Washington would expose Blue's weaknesses as a leader.

When the war was over, Congress saddled his agency with the responsibility of caring for returning veterans, but gave it few funds with which to fulfill its new mandate. More than 200,000 wounded and disabled veterans came back from Europe, overwhelming the Service's ability to provide treatment. Blue ordered rush conversions of underused quarantine stations into veterans' hospitals, satisfying no one. Complaints about the patchwork system funneled into Washington and continued to grow louder, undercutting the political capital Blue had acquired. He further distanced himself from power by pushing for an education campaign warning the public that returning soldiers could spread venereal disease. Though medically responsible, it was canceled by President Woodrow Wilson, a prim former college professor who took office in 1916 after a long career focused on extolling the influence of the Puritans on American culture.

Distracted by his responsibility to provide care for veterans, Blue neglected the original mandate of the Public Health Service. An outbreak of a deadly strain of influenza, known as the Spanish flu, emerged in March 1918 and spread quickly across the country. The disease, the first serious flu epidemic to emerge in the United States in more than twenty-five years, seemed to prey upon young, healthy adults, as if intent on erasing a generation.

The speed at which the disease traveled made it seem like the very air was infected. On September 7, one of the forty-five thousand soldiers stationed at Camp Devens, an Army training base on the outskirts of Boston, reported to the base's hospital. Staff observed that the man seemed delirious and diagnosed him with meningitis, and he joined the approximately ninety other patients then under care at a hospital designed to hold up to 1,200. The next day, a dozen more soldiers appeared with the same symptoms. More and more sick men began appearing, prompting doctors to change their diagnosis to influenza. At the peak of the outbreak, 1,543 soldiers at the base fell ill in a single day. With so many doctors and workers sick that there was no one left to provide care, the hospital stopped accepting new patients, leaving soldiers to die in their barracks.

"These men start with what appears to be an ordinary attack of LaGrippe or Influenza, and when brought to the Hosp. they very rapidly develop the most vicious type of Pneumonia that has ever been seen. Two hours after admission they have the Mahogany spots over the cheek bones, and a few hours later you can begin to see the Cyanosis [a term for a patient turning blue from lack of oxygen]," wrote Roy Grist, a physician at the hospital. "It is only a matter of a few hours then until death comes . . . It is horrible. . . . We have been averaging about 100 deaths per day . . . For several days there were no coffins and the bodies piled up something fierce."

By October, the Public Health Service was tracking thousands of deaths a week from the flu. Up to 40 percent of service members in the Army and Navy developed symptoms, crippling the nation's ability to protect itself. Shipyards up and down the East Coast had to close for days at a time because there weren't enough healthy workers. In San Antonio, 53 percent of the city's population came down with the disease; in Philadelphia, twelve thousand people died within a six-week span. Families began to fear their relatives; neighbors saw in every cough the germs that would lead to their own deaths. Philadelphia's head of emergency aid begged, "We simply must have more volunteer helpers . . . these people are almost all at the point of death." In Kentucky a Red Cross official reported that there were "hundreds of cases . . . [of infected] people starving to death not from lack of food but because the well were panic stricken and would not go near the sick." Victor Vaughn, the head of the Army's communicable disease division, wrote in his diary that "If the epidemic continues its mathematical rate of acceleration, civilization could easily disappear . . . from the face of the earth within a matter of a few more weeks."

Blue was slow to respond to the epidemic, wasting weeks as his officers tried to get samples of the bacterium from different areas of the country to see if it was the same strain that had caused widespread deaths in 1893. Unlike the plague, which could be tracked by the movement patterns of rats, the flu spread as if at random, frustrating any attempt to contain it. As the death toll rose, Blue continued to downplay the significance of the outbreak. In May of

1918, Congress had passed the Sedition Act, levying prison terms of up to twenty years for spreading information that interfered with the country's war effort. Officers at all levels of government focused on maintaining the country's morale while suppressing information that undercut Americans' sense of safety. "There is no cause for alarm if precautions are observed," Blue told reporters, though he knew otherwise. His few public instructions to combat the disease included reminders of the importance of washing hands with soap and water and avoiding crowded places, especially if one was already feeling ill. The advice made little impact, and over the last three months of 1918 more than four million Americans were infected with the disease, causing 400,000 fatalities and dropping the average American life span by twelve years. Among pregnant women, fatality rates ranged from 23 percent to 71 percent.

The third wave of the flu began in January of 1919. Among its victims was President Wilson, who collapsed while attending the Versailles Peace Conference. His fever climbed to 103 degrees and he suffered intense coughing fits, leaving him in such a weak and confused state that it was widely commented upon by other attendees. A young aide accompanying the president to Paris died after coming down with similar symptoms. Wilson struggled throughout the proceedings, and his diminished capacities were later seen as one of the reasons why the Treasury of Versailles, which ended the First World War, was so deeply flawed. The harsh penalties it imposed on Germany helped fuel Hitler's rise to power.

Then, as quickly as the flu appeared, it vanished, its lethal power subdued as those who had been exposed to earlier waves developed immunity. The disease killed an estimated 675,000 Americans, ten times as many as died in the war. Between fifty and one hundred million people died worldwide, with the most deaths concentrated in areas far from medical care. In the Fiji Islands, 14 percent of the population died within sixteen days; in some areas of Alaska, entire villages developed the disease and perished within the span of a week.

Though it was impossible to ignore the failure of the Public Health Service to stop the disease, Blue assumed that the end of the pandemic would allow him to return to his primary mission of improving the nation's sanitary conditions. His four-year term was scheduled to expire in 1920, and he wrote an eleven-page memorandum in March of 1919 outlining the goals he intended to accomplish over the next four years. Among other plans, he proposed to expand the so-called "pure milk" laws to require pasteurization nationwide, establish clinics for sick children and implement a form of national health insurance.

He had little inkling that politics would intervene. On the morning of October 2, President Wilson suffered a stroke that left him paralyzed on his left side and blind in his right eye. Wilson's wife, Edith, conspired with his personal physician, Dr. Cary T. Grayson, to hide the president's condition from the country for the remainder of his term. With Edith Wilson effectively serving as the nation's chief executive, the Wilson administration leaned heavily on trusted allies in Washington. Treasury Secretary Carter Glass soon began lobbying to replace Blue with Hugh Cummings, a twenty-five-year veteran of the Public Health Service who hailed from Glass's home state of Virginia and who carried none of the baggage from the poor treatment of returning veterans or the country's ill-equipped response to the flu. Edith Wilson offered no objections and signed off on the plan.

Blue thus became the first Surgeon General in the country's history who was involuntary removed from office. Not knowing what else to do with his life at the age of fifty-two, he accepted a demotion and continued to serve in a lower role, all the while growing increasingly bitter. Eager to keep his deposed rival away from power, Glass sent Blue on a series of assignments in Europe which kept him outside the U.S. for several years. Blue's work in bringing modern sanitation methods to France earned him the Legion of Honor in 1923, fulfilling a dream that he had nursed as a child on the cotton fields of South Carolina. "You will recall that as a boy I admired the

First Napoleon perhaps more than any other figure in history, and that I never tired of reading his life and of his deeds as a soldier and as a statesman," he wrote in a letter to his sister Kate after receiving the award. "I never thought then that I would ever receive, much less deserve, the decoration which he bestowed upon his officers and men . . . I wear the ribbon in the lapels of all my coats."

Though it helped restore his self-worth, the award was not enough to soothe the resentment that had built up toward not only his replacement but other men in the Service whom he considered disloyal. Blue began drinking heavily and was known to start listing all the slights and sins he had suffered, calling his rivals "snakes" and "damned skunks." One night, he turned his wrath on Rucker, who had served next to him in San Francisco and New Orleans faithfully, calling him a "God-dam apostate." The insult stung Rucker and they did not speak again for years.

At an age when many men were considering retirement, Blue felt alone. He had long ago accepted that he would remain single for his entire life, without a family of his own to turn to. Yet the Service had always provided him something that he had ached for as a boy: a purpose. Now that too was gone, and there seemed to be nothing left to redeem him.

CHAPTER 18

A HERO ONCE MORE

On October 2, 1924, a physician named Giles Porter pulled up outside a small home at 700 Clara Street, a few blocks away from the Los Angeles River. The sun hung high overhead in the empty blue sky, giving no indication that autumn was approaching. The city's obliviousness to the changing of the seasons was a large part of what had drawn more than a million new residents to Los Angeles over the last two decades, creating what was at the time the nation's fifth-largest metropolis with a sprawl of broad streets lined with young palm trees.

Clara Street belonged to an older, poorer Los Angeles. Less than half a mile away stood the Los Angeles Plaza, the site where the city had been officially founded in 1781 as little more than a trading post amid the empty valleys of Southern California. The neighborhood remained rooted in its Spanish past even as the city changed around it. Well-to-do white immigrants fleeing the harsh winters of the East Coast settled first in English-speaking districts to the west of nearby Union Station, the region's chief link with the rest of the country, and expanded outward from there, filling in some of the nation's first suburbs.

What remained in the neighborhood surrounding Clara Street

were the remnants of a forgotten era that had not yet been wiped away. Olvera, one of the oldest streets in the city, was less than a ten-minute walk away, and along its muddy alleyway stood the Avila Adobe, built by one of the first Mexican mayors of Los Angeles when it was a village home to fewer than five hundred people. The building, which had served as headquarters for Commodore Robert Stockton and General Stephen W. Kearny when they captured the city during the Mexican American War, was now run down and dilapidated, buffeted on all sides by machine shops and grime. Tracks leading into Union Station were close enough that passing trains rattled dishes and forced a temporary pause in conversation, the future once again imposing itself upon the past.

As he got out of the car, Porter could see downtown Los Angeles rising behind him, where workers were clearing a lot on Spring Street in advance of the construction of a new thirty-two-story City Hall that when completed, would be topped by a soaring white tower jutting into the sky like a monument to progress. He walked up to the door and knocked, not sure of what he would find. Inside, Jesús Lajun lay suffering from what appeared to be the flu. A laborer fo the Los Angeles streetcar system, Lajun had missed the last few da of work with a high fever, and swollen lymph nodes along his thi and groin made it difficult for him to move. His fifteen-year daughter, Francisca, lay nearby, overcome by what appeared to b same virus. Porter saw nothing remarkable about their conditio told them to rest, leaving the home not long after he had ente

Francisca's symptoms worsened the next day. A thirty-nin old neighbor named Luciana Samarano, then six months p offered to stay at the house to care for her until she recove girl's fever seemed immune to any remedy, prompting Je to call for an ambulance on October 4. Francisca died c to the hospital, due to what doctors on call listed as dc monia. Jesús, still ill, remained at home, where his fev to climb. He died one week after his daughter from said was pneumonia.

Over the following days, others on Clara Street came down with what seemed to be a particularly lethal form of the disease. A physician by the name of George Stevens called Los Angeles General Hospital to report that he had cared for several patients in the neighborhood who all complained of chest pains, backache, fever and a deep, hacking cough. The quick onset of symptoms was like no form of pneumonia that he had seen before, he warned hospital staff, leaving him puzzled as to whether it might be a different, more deadly illness.

Ten days after she cared for the dying girl in the Lajun household, Luciana Samarano fell ill. She sequestered herself in a back room at 742 Clara Street, a small single-story house that she shared with her family and a few boarders, and hoped that the illness would pass. On October 19, she suffered a miscarriage and died a few hours later, having never broken her fever. Doctors who arrived to issue a death certificate saw nothing unusual and allowed the body to remain in the home, where the Samarano family held a funeral service before burial.

Soon other members of her family became sick, as if they were the next ones standing in a line of dominoes. Her husband, Guadalupe Samarano, developed a fever in the days following Luciana's funeral and quickly deteriorated. His weakened condition prompted his family to call a priest, Father Medrano Brualla from Our Lady Queen of Angels Church, to administer last rites before an ambulance arrived and took him to General Hospital. He died the same afternoon and his body was released to his family, who once again held a funeral service at home.

In the following days, nearly everyone who had attended the funeral fell ill. Father Brualla, who spoke at both funerals, was rushed to General Hospital where he died before doctors could stabilize him. The four Samarano brothers, ranging in age from ten-year-old Roberto to eighteen-month-old Raúl, arrived at the same hospital after developing the same high fever and deep, painful cough that had killed their parents.

Fearing an outbreak of meningitis, doctors took tissue samples not only from the Samarano boys but from dozens of other patients who began appearing at the hospital with the same symptoms, all of them arriving from within the blocks of Clara Street. Dr. George Maner, the hospital pathologist, joked with a colleague that this was what an outbreak of plague must look like. He then peered through a microscope at a biopsy taken from Roberto Samarano's body and discovered that it was teeming with pneumonic plague, the most virulent form of the disease. He stood up, white-faced, and asked a doctor nearby to take a look, though there was no need. The distinctive rod-shaped bacilli were obvious, a part of the rudimentary training in bacteriology that every doctor now received. Suddenly the wave of deaths made sense and pointed to an inescapable conclusion: after more than a decade in remission, plague had returned to kill again.

Over the next several hours, the assistant superintendent of the hospital sent telegrams to federal and state officials and medical supply dealers throughout the state, asking if any doses of plague serum were available. The request piqued the interest of Benjamin Brown, a Public Health Service surgeon stationed in Los Angeles, who arrived unannounced at General Hospital and quickly confirmed his suspicions. He wired Surgeon General Cummings in code that afternoon, noting "Eighteen cases ekkil [pneumonic plague]. Three suspects. Ten begs [deaths]. Ethos [situation bad]. Recommend federal aid."

Police began stringing rope around the eight blocks surrounding Macy Street, the nearest main thoroughfare to Clara Street, shortly after one on the morning of November 2. Approximately 2,500 residents, the vast majority of them Mexican American, were sealed into quarantine. Seven-day rations were given to each household while health officers accompanied by a Spanish-speaking interpreter began a house-to-house inspection in search of additional carriers of the disease. Anyone who lived in the same building as a known plague victim was taken to General Hospital as a precaution, cloistering 114 potential cases in a handful of rooms.

Those who remained in the district were told to wear thick clothing at all times and urged to clean their homes as thoroughly as they could. Policemen patrolled the edges of the district, preventing anyone from entering or leaving. Shortly after sunrise, Nora Sterry, the white principal of an elementary school in the neighborhood, was turned away. "They can't keep me out," she vowed to reporters who had gathered at the quarantine lines. "All my children are in there. And, if you see the flag waving from the mast in the Macy Street schoolyard tomorrow morning, you will know I am there." Indeed, the flag rose the next morning. Sterry, with the help of two missionaries, turned the school's cafeteria into a relief station, cooking food for families whose rations were already running low.

Fear of the disease spread throughout the city, fueled in part by the refusal of the press to confirm or deny its presence. The *Los Angeles Times*, the dominant newspaper in the city—which considered boosting Southern California as a land of sunshine and happiness its most important function—waited until the sixth day of the quarantine to identify the disease as plague, which it insisted was only "the technical term for the malignant pneumonia appearing in a small area of the Mexican quarter." Others in the city acted more quickly. The newly opened Biltmore Hotel, then the largest hotel west of Chicago, fired all of the 150 Latino workers on its staff regardless of whether they lived near the infected district. Walter Dickie, the secretary of the state Board of Health, urged the city and the Chamber of Commerce to "insist that all of that area where Mexicans live is put in sanitary condition and undoubtedly there is a great deal of that area that ought to be condemned and destroyed." Four other predominantly Latino neighborhoods were soon placed under quarantine, though no new victims had been found.

By the middle of November forty people were dead from plague, all of them in some way connected to Luciana Samarano. The trail of victims included her mother, sister, uncle, husband, three of her sons, her stepmother, a stepbrother, four friends, five cousins, six boarders, a nurse who treated her, the nurse's sister, the priest who administered last rites to her husband, the ambulance driver who drove her husband to the hospital and a neighbor. They died within a span of two weeks, their burials proceeding like a grim parade. All had died after developing the pneumonic form of the disease, which can be spread merely by a cough. Hoping to forestall a wider epidemic, health officials burned down the Samarano home and every other residence that had harbored the victims. Then they waited, hoping that no new cases would emerge.

In interviews with surviving residents of Clara Street, investigators learned that in the week before his death Jesús Lajun had laughed when describing the difficulty he had in removing the putrid body of a dead rat he had discovered underneath his house. The animal had long since been disposed of, but it gave health officials their first clue. It appeared that the strain of plague that by now was endemic among squirrels in Northern California had finally arrived in Los Angeles. City officials announced an eradication program targeting rats and squirrels, following the methods set down by Rupert Blue in San Francisco some twenty years before.

The only question was who would lead the cleanup. Just as in San Francisco nearly twenty-five years earlier, the city, state and Public Health Service had competing claims of jurisdiction, and each sought the glory—and funding—that would come with taking responsibility for eliminating the outbreak. After the state Board of Health refused to allow Public Health Service members to take part in the eradication effort, Surgeon General Cummings declared the port of Los Angeles plague-infected, forcing all departing vessels to fly a quarantine flag and await inspection at subsequent harbors. The head of the city's Chamber of Commerce sent a letter to Washington calling the move "ridiculous" and an unnecessary threat to the state's economy given that the outbreak of the disease occurred some twenty-two miles from the port.

In hopes of defusing the standoff, the director of the state Board of Health invited Cummings to travel to Los Angeles to see the conditions for himself. He quickly agreed. "I have always felt that if we could get together we could straighten out what appeared to be a rather awkward situation," Cummings wrote. "My only purpose has been to assist the state in getting rid of this condition quickly."

The tour accomplished little. Cummings returned to Washington still livid that the Service had not been formally asked to take over the rat eradication program, which, if done, would have prompted Congress to increase its annual appropriation. City and state legislators, meanwhile, tried to pass the responsibility of paying for the cleanup efforts to each other. After the City Council slashed sanitation funding in an attempt to force the state's hand, Mayor George Cryer sent a formal letter to President Calvin Coolidge requesting that the Public Health Service take over. Though he was now finally in control over the cleanup campaign, Cummings felt pressure from the White House to quickly remedy the situation. Any misstep could escalate into a national embarrassment, undermining his tenure in office. Boxed in by politics, he was forced to turn to the one man he knew could accomplish the job.

For the last decade, Cummings had kept Rupert Blue far away from Washington and any high-profile roles in the Service so as not to feel threatened by the man he had displaced. At the time of the plague outbreak in Los Angeles, Blue had just returned from an international conference in Switzerland devoted to the growing narcotics trade and was preparing for a routine tour of medical facilities in the Midwest. Instead, his new orders in hand, he once again boarded a train for California, intent on completing the mission he had started as a young man.

He arrived in a place he barely recognized. Los Angeles was now the largest city in the state and growing larger, replacing San Francisco as the primary destination for newcomers. The greatest concentration of automobiles in the country glided along its maze of streets, across a geography that stretched from the ocean to mountains to the edge of the desert. The year before Blue arrived, Harry Chandler, the publisher of the *Los Angeles Times*, erected thirteen letters, each thirty feet wide and forty-three feet tall, atop Mount Lee as a way to publicize his upscale real estate development high in the hills. When illuminated by light boxes situated below each letter, the Hollywoodland sign glowed across the Los Angeles basin each night, a beacon for hundreds who arrived by bus and train each day intent on becoming a star. Among them was a young cartoonist from Kansas City named Walt Disney, who had stepped off a train the summer before with forty dollars and a one-reel cartoon from his bankrupt company in a cardboard suitcase.

The city's expanding industry of glamour was foreign to a man who had grown to fear the spotlight. Blue, now fifty-six and his muscular frame but a memory, still felt the scars of failure from the Spanish flu outbreak six years earlier. Though he had traveled around the globe and won accolades in the succeeding years, he could not shake the pain of doubt, regretting that he had not done more when he had the chance. The reemergence of plague gave him an opportunity to feel useful one more time, if only to remind himself of the good that he had been able to accomplish in the past.

Blue began implementing the same rodent control measures he had developed in San Francisco and New Orleans. Houses in the Clara Street neighborhood were stripped of their siding to prevent rats from building nests; garbage collection was increased, starving the animals of food; poison was applied liberally throughout the city and along the wharves. Blue sent teams of men into the rural expanses of Los Angeles County searching for squirrel holes, which they dynamited and poisoned. Property owners were ordered to spend what soon amounted to more than $2 million on retrofitting their buildings with concrete, razing the few remaining wooden structures which survived as relics of the city's past.

Blue stayed in Los Angeles for several months, thrilled to feel a sense of purpose in his life again. The irony that his replacement as

Surgeon General had been forced to turn to him in a time of crisis was not lost on him, though he did not voice it. He was too happy to once again be attacking the disease which had slipped through his fingers and reached the open expanses of Northern California. He considered his time in Los Angeles an act of retribution, and would not allow himself to rest until the danger from the disease had passed.

By the end of the year, health officers under his supervision had sliced open the bodies of 106,951 rats, finding 187 that tested positive for plague. An additional 16,094 squirrels passed through Blue's laboratory, with nine of them infected by the disease. No new human victims were found, capping the city's pain at Clara Street. Yet Blue remained wary, considering it only a matter of time before plague struck again. In his annual report, Surgeon General Cummings noted that the Service would have to remain ready to battle the disease. "I have no doubt that, under present conditions, this squirrel infection will continue for many years to come," he wrote. "This reservoir of plague in the United States should ever be kept in mind, nor should our vigilance in maintaining squirrel-free zones around rat-infested cities in these infected counties be relaxed."

Los Angeles would prove to be the last major outbreak of plague in the country. After helping eradicate the disease from the city, Blue continued his nomadic work in the Service on assignments designed by Cummings to keep him busy. His nephews often wrote him letters, gently suggesting that he retire from roaming the globe and settle down someplace warm like Florida. Ever tactful, Blue respectfully ignored their advice and continued on the only path of life he had ever known until 1932, when advancing heart disease forced him to retire from the Service at the age of sixty-four. He maintained a small room in a hotel in Washington, unable to the end to settle down into the familiar trappings of a home of his own. He died on April 12, 1948, one month shy of his eightieth birthday, at a hospital in Charleston. His body was taken home to Marion, where it was laid to rest in a grave next to his sisters Kate and Henriette.

Under a canopy of Spanish moss, his gravestone now rises above the South Carolina soil, the emblem of the Public Health Service etched into its face. The Service allowed him to fulfill every dream that he had had as a young boy playing in the nearby cotton fields, and even some that once seemed impossible. He had traveled the world in the service of others, advised the powerful and helped save the lives of hundreds, if not millions, of people. His career began in a quarantine station treating passengers who came aboard steamships, and by its end he was protecting travelers riding aboard jet planes. He rose to the highest peaks of his profession and, after politics robbed him of his status, rose again to become a hero once more. Yet above the body of the man whose work saved millions of lives stands only a simple inscription: "His work for humanity took him to many lands but he came home to sleep his long last sleep."

HOW CLOSE WE CAME

There are few reminders of the fight to save America from plague or how close it came to devastating the country. The men and women who played a role in confronting the disease scattered across the country, leaving the horror of what they had seen behind.

Joseph Kinyoun, the man whose presence was enough to cause riots in San Francisco, worked for several private companies after resigning from the Marine Hospital Service and eventually became a professor at George Washington University. He died in 1919, his reputation having never recovered. As part of its 125-year anniversary in 2012, the National Institutes of Health recognized him as its "forgotten forefather," tracing its history back to the laboratory he founded on Staten Island. Governor Henry Gage, the man who essentially ran Kinyoun out of California, returned to private law practice when his party refused to renominate him for office and died in Los Angeles in August 1924, just two months before that city faced its own outbreak of the disease that he had refused to acknowledge. James D. Phelan, the mayor of San Francisco during the initial outbreak, went on to represent California in the U.S. Senate from 1915 to 1921, where he continued to advocate banning all immigration from Asia. In May 2017, the University of San Francisco removed his name from a student residence hall and renamed it in honor of Burl Toler, a graduate of the university who went on to become both the first African American official in a major American professional sports league and the first black secondary school principal in San Francisco history.

Colby Rucker, who served as Blue's closest confidant in San Francisco and New Orleans, died in 1930 after an insect bite suffered on a golf course in Louisiana became infected. Victor Blue, Rupert's imposingly successful older brother, retired from the Navy as a rear admiral in 1919 and died in 1928. The USS *Blue*, a destroyer, was dedicated by Kate Lilly Blue at the Norfolk Navy Yard in 1937. The ship became part of the Pacific Fleet and was in port at Pearl Harbor when Japanese planes launched a surprise attack on December 7, 1941. The ship made it safely out to sea with only four junior officers aboard and spent months protecting convoys between Hawaii and San Francisco before taking part in the Battle of Guadalcanal. The ship was torpedoed by a Japanese destroyer and sunk on August 23, 1942.

Angel Island, where Kinyoun was banished by a vengeful Surgeon General and made the first positive identification of plague in the United States, became an immigration center in 1910, and over the following three decades saw more than one million people pass through what is now called the "Ellis Island of the West." It is now a popular state park, flush with mountain bikers and the scent of barbecues on weekends. The intersection of Jackson Street and Grant Avenue, where the body of the first victim of the plague was found in the Globe Hotel, now features a Citibank and competing discount clothing stores. It is still in the heart of San Francisco's Chinatown, which remains the world's most densely populated Chinatown outside Asia and one of the most popular tourist attractions in the city. Sadly, records of the lives of its plague survivors are hard to come by, leaving the full stories of those who experienced the terror of quarantine and prejudice untold.

In Los Angeles, the plague-infected homes along Clara Street were never rebuilt. The site of the city's outbreak now falls under the shadow of the Twin Towers Correctional Facility, which was the world's largest jail at the time of its construction and after a series of scandals now holds the county's mentally ill prisoner population. A three-story brick building, the home of a bail bond company, stands at the approximate location of the Samarano home, across the street from a lone palm tree. Olvera Street and the surrounding neighborhood has been remade into a tourist attraction celebrating the city's Mexican heritage. Our Lady Queen of Angels Catholic church, the pastoral home of Father Medrano Brualla, still stands overlooking Los Angeles Plaza, where a fleet of food trucks congregate every weekend.

Plague has never been fully eradicated from the country. The strain of the disease that first infected squirrels in the hills above Berkeley was carried by fleas deeper into the continent, eventually becoming entrenched in rodent populations throughout the West as a permanent reminder of how politics and circumstances conspired to prevent Blue from containing the plague when he had a chance. Two visitors to Yosemite National Park developed plague in the summer of 2015, while multiple patients developed the disease in Arizona and New Mexico in the summer of 2017.

An average of seven people in the United States now contract plague each year, according to the Centers for Disease Control, with a multiyear high of seventeen cases occurring in 2006. Patients whose conditions would have quickly proven fatal are now treated with antibiotics such as streptomycin that were unavailable in Blue's time. The continued usage of such drugs worries some researchers, who fear that the plague bacterium may evolve to become drug-resistant, making the disease untreatable once more. In the meantime, the disease remains hidden along the wide open horizon of the West, where it waits to once again make a jump into the human population.

ACKNOWLEDGMENTS

This book began with an angry letter written by a homesick man.

Frederick Rindge, one of the main characters in my last book, was once one of the wealthiest people in California, and owned all the land that makes up what is now the city of Malibu. As part of maintaining a business empire that stretched from Los Angeles to Boston to South America, he regularly traveled north to San Francisco. In a letter to his wife, May, he wrote that he had heard rumors that plague was in the city, a place he called "the wickedest place I ever saw."

I grew up in California, once lived in the Bay Area, and am the kind of person who stops to read historical markers, yet I had never heard of anyone contracting plague in California, much less dying from it. My research propelled me into an alternative history, in which a disease capable of killing millions not only arrived in San Francisco but stayed there for years, threatening the entire country.

I am deeply indebted to the many people who helped me turn that discovery into the book you are now holding.

I was fortunate to find several researchers with connections to the story who were kind enough to share their expertise with me. Dr. David Morens of the U.S. Public Health Service and Dr. Victoria Harden and Barbara Faye Hawkins, both of the National Institutes of Health, pointed me to documents and letters detailing the life of Joseph Kinyoun and patiently answered my questions about the history of bacteriology and public health. Dr. Guenter B. Risse, professor emeritus at the University of California, San Francisco, not only wrote the definitive history of the Chinatown plague but helped point me in the right direction for materials and responded to all my queries quickly. John Rees at the National Library of Medicine helped me track down several letters and research papers written by Kinyoun, as well as speeches made at his farewell party in Washington before he was exiled to the West Coast.

J. Michael Hughes trusted me with dozens of original copies of letters written by Rupert Blue, helping me get a deeper sense of his personality, as well as photographs of Blue throughout his lifetime.

The immensely talented team at W. W. Norton once again made publishing a book far easier than it should be. My wonderful editor, Jill Bialosky, championed the project from the get-go and helped me go deeper into the story. Allegra Huston, my brilliant copyeditor, saved me from several embarrassing mistakes. Special thanks also go to Bill Rusin, for his early enthusiasm, and Drew Weitman, who shepherded the manuscript along its way to publication, as well as Josie Freedman at ICM Partners.

My agents, Larry Weissman and Sascha Alper, helped shape this book from the beginning and remain two of the most generous people that I know.

Alan Yang, Jennifer Ablan, Lauren Young, Helen Coster, Matthew Craft, John and Carol Ordover, Tony and Maryanne Petrizio, Robert and Gina Scott, and Ryan and Diane Randall all offered advice, guidance and support throughout this project.

And finally, infinite love and thanks go to Megan, Henry, and Isla Randall, without whom none of this would be possible.

SELECTED BIBLIOGRAPHY

Sources are listed in the order in which they inform the text.

PROLOGUE: FIGHTING THE DEVIL WITH FIRE

Mohr, James. *Plague and Fire: Battling Black Death and the 1900 Burning of Honolulu's Chinatown.* New York: Oxford University Press, 2005.

Bonner, John. "Questions of the Day." *California Illustrated Magazine* 5, 1893.

Li, Ling-Ai. *Life is For a Long Time: A Chinese Hawaiian Memoir.* New York: Hastings House, 1972.

Burlingame, Burl. "The City at War." *Honolulu Star–Bulletin,* January 31, 2000.

Cantor, Norman. *In the Wake of the Plague: The Black Death and the World It Made.* New York: Simon & Schuster, 2001.

Kelly, John. *The Great Mortality: An Intimate History of the Black Death, the Most Devastating Plague of All Time.* New York: Harper Collins, 2005.

CHAPTER 1: ACROSS THE SEA

Letters of Joseph J. Kinyoun. History of Medicine Division, National Library of Medicine, Bethesda, MD.

Kobe, George M. "Complimentary Dinner to Joseph J. Kinyoun, M.D., Ph.D., Given on the Occasion of His Departure for San Francisco, Cal., by the Members of the Medical Profession, Washington, D.C." Reprinted in *The Georgetown College Journal,* June 1899.

Arena, Eva. "Taming Dreaded Diseases in the 1800s: Joseph Kinyoun, the Hygienic Laboratory, and the Origins of the NIH." *The NIH Catalyst.* 20, no. 6 (November–December 2012).

Morens, David M., and Anthony S. Fauci. "The Forgotten Forefather: Joseph James Kinyoun and the Founding of the National Institutes of Health." *MBio* 3, no. 4 (June 2012).

CHAPTER 2: THE *NIPPON MARU*

Annual Report of the Supervising Surgeon-General of the Marine-Hospital Service of the United States for the Fiscal Year 1899. Washington: Government Printing Office, 1901.

"Bubonic Plague on the Nippon Maru." *San Francisco Chronicle*, June 26, 1899.

"Two Bodies off a Plague Ship." *San Francisco Chronicle*, June 27, 1899.

"The Plague in Politics." *San Francisco Chronicle*, June 28, 1899.

"Wyman Knows of No Plague." *San Francisco Chronicle*, June 28, 1899.

"Quarantine Is At Least Raised." *San Francisco Chronicle*, June 29, 1899.

"Germs and Politics: Two Kinds of Bacilli in the Plague Scare." *San Francisco Chronicle*, June 30, 1899.

"Child of the Quarantine." *San Francisco Chronicle*, July 5, 1899.

"It Was Not the Plague." *San Francisco Chronicle*, July 1, 1899.

"Health Board in Bad Light." *San Francisco Chronicle*, July 3, 1899.

Mohr, James. *Plague and Fire: Battling Black Death and the 1900 Burning of Honolulu's Chinatown.* New York: Oxford University Press, 2005.

CHAPTER 3: THE IMPERIAL CITY

Sutter, John. "The Discovery of Gold in California." *Hutchins' California Magazine*, November 1857. Accessed via the Virtual Museum of the City of San Francisco at http://www.sfmuseum.org/hist2/gold.html.

Platt, James. *Platt's Essays.* Vol. 1. London: Simpkin, Marshall, and Co., 1883.

Albertsson, Dean. "The Discovery of Gold in California as Viewed by New York and London." *The Pacific Spectator* 3, no. 1 (Winter 1949). Accessed via the Virtual Museum of the City of San Francisco at http://www.sfmuseum.org/hist5/albertson.html.

"The Gold Hunter's Farewell to His Wife." *Illinois State Journal*, February 21, 1849. Accessed via the Virtual Museum of the City of San Francisco at http://www.sfmuseum.org/hist7/poem2.html.

Starr, Kevin, and Richard J. Orsi, eds. *Rooted in Barbarous Soil: People, Culture, and Community in Gold Rush California.* Berkeley: University of California Press, 2000.

Marks, Paula Mitchell. *Precious Dust: The Saga of the Western Gold Rushes.* New York: William Morrow, 1994.

Field, Stephen J. *Personal Reminiscences of Early Days in California, With Other Sketches.* Privately published, 1893.

"Barbary Coast 1887, An Odd Corner of San Francisco." *San Francisco News Letter*, May 7, 1887. Accessed via the Virtual Museum of San Francisco at http://www .sfmuseum.org/hist12/barbarycoast.html.

George, Henry. "What the Railroad Will Bring Us." *Overland Monthly* 1, no. 4 (October, 1868).

Nolte, Carl. "The Death of the Imperial City." *San Francisco Chronicle*, April 18, 1999.

Irwin, Will. *The City That Was*. New York: B. W. Huebsch, 1908.

Chase, Marilyn. *The Barbary Plague*. New York: Random House, 2003.

Barnett, John. "Report of the Bureau of Building Condition of City Hall." Accessed via the Virtual Museum of San Francisco at http://www.sfmuseum .org/hist1/repairs.html.

Jordan, David Starr. *California and the Californians and the Alps of King–Kern Divide*. San Francisco: The Whitaker–Ray Company, 1903.

Craddock, Susan. *City of Plagues: Disease, Poverty and Deviance in San Francisco*. Minneapolis: University of Minnesota Press, 2000.

Keevak, Michael. *Becoming Yellow: A Short History of Racial Thinking*. Princeton, NJ: Princeton University Press, 2011.

Bancroft, Hubert Howe. *The Works of Hubert Howe Bancroft*. Volume XXXVIII. San Francisco: The History Company, 1890.

Chinese Railroad Workers in North America Project at Stanford University. Accessed at http://web.stanford.edu/group/chineserailroad/cgi-bin/wordpress/.

Wallace, Kelly. "Forgotten Los Angeles History: The Chinese Massacre of 1871." Los Angeles Public Library, May 19, 2017. Accessed at https://www.lapl.org/ collections-resources/blogs/lapl/chinese-massacre-1871.

"Remarks by Mr. Denis Kearney on Kearneyism in California." *American Commonwealth* 2 (1899). Accessed via the Virtual Museum of San Francisco at http:// www.sfmuseum.net/hist9/brycenotes.html.

Phelan, James. "The Ideal San Francisco." *San Francisco News Letter*, 1897. Accessed via the Virtual Museum of California at http://www.sfmuseum.org/hist5/ ideal.html.

Risse, Guenter B. *Plague, Fear, and Politics in San Francisco's Chinatown*. Baltimore: Johns Hopkins University Press, 2012.

CHAPTER 4: CRIMINAL IDIOCY

"Health Board is Forced to Abandon Its Bubonic Bluff." *San Francisco Chronicle*, March 10, 1900.

Risse, Guenter B. *Plague, Fear, and Politics in San Francisco's Chinatown*. Baltimore: Johns Hopkins University Press, 2012.

"May Not Prove an Unmixed Evil." *San Francisco Chronicle*, January 3, 1900.

"Not Much Alarmed by the Plague." *San Francisco Chronicle*, January 4, 1900.

"The Bubonic Plague." *San Francisco Chronicle*, January 9, 1900.

"At Work on Serum to Cure the Plague." *San Francisco Chronicle*, January 28, 1900.

"Abate the Nuisances." *San Francisco Chronicle*, February 24, 1900.

"Put a Block on the Chinese Quarter." *San Francisco Chronicle*, March 7, 1900.

"Nothing but a Suspicion: Criminal Idiocy of the Phelan Health Board." *San Francisco Chronicle*, March 8, 1900.

"Plague Fake Is Exposed." *San Francisco Chronicle*, March 9, 1900.

"Police Keeping Quarantine Guard over Chinatown." *San Francisco Call*, March 7, 1900.

"Chinatown Quarantined." *San Francisco Call*, March 8, 1900.

Wright, Arnold. *Twentieth Century Impressions of Hong Kong, Shanghai, and other Treasury Ports of China: Their History, People, Commerce, Industries and Resources*. London: Lloyd's Greater Britain Publishing Company, 1908.

Bibel, David J., and T. H. Chen. "Diagnosis of Plague: An Analysis of the Yersin–Kitasato Controversy. *Bacteriological Reviews*, September 1976.

Hawgood, Barbara J. "Alexandre Yersin (1863–1943): discoverer of the plague bacillus, explorer and agronomist." *Journal of Medical Biography* 16, no. 3 (August 1, 2008).

"The Plague a Phantom." *San Francisco Chronicle*, March 13, 1900.

"No Plague Is Found: Fruitless Efforts of the Medical Inspectors in Chinatown." *San Francisco Chronicle*, March 14, 1900.

"Bubonic Scare Has Collapsed." *San Francisco Chronicle*, March 17, 1900.

Letters of Joseph J. Kinyoun. History of Medicine Division, National Library of Medicine, Bethesda, MD.

CHAPTER 5: FAULT LINES

Annual Report of the Supervising Surgeon-General of the Marine-Hospital Service of the United States for the Fiscal Year 1899. Washington: Government Printing Office, 1901.

"Pegging Away at the Plague: Health Board Bent on Making a Scare." *San Francisco Chronicle*, March 21, 1900.

"Health Board Brings Calamity on this City." *San Francisco Chronicle*, March 22, 1900.

"Found Not a Single Germ: Phelan's Health Board Hunting for Plague." *San Francisco Chronicle*, March 23, 1900.

"Health Gang Wants Cash." *San Francisco Chronicle*, March 25, 1900.

"A Crime Against Trade Interests." *San Francisco Chronicle*, April 2, 1900.

"No Bubonic Plague in San Francisco." *San Francisco Call*, April 3, 1900.

"What Plagues Us." *San Francisco Call*, April 3, 1900.

"Should Suffer for the Plague." *San Francisco Call*, April 4, 1900.

"Serious Charges Made." *San Francisco Chronicle*, April 5, 1900.

"Deprecate Plague Fake." *San Francisco Chronicle*, April 17, 1900.

"Results of Fake Plague Spread by Examiner–Journal." *San Francisco Call*, April 11, 1900.

"State Medicos Dined." *San Francisco Call*, April 20, 1900.

"Submit Proofs or Retract." *San Francisco Call*, May 24, 1900.

"Editorial." *San Francisco Call*, April 8, 1900.

Hoy, Suellen. *Chasing Dirt: The American Pursuit of Cleanliness*. New York: Oxford University Press, 1995.

Risse, Guenter B. *Plague, Fear, and Politics in San Francisco's Chinatown*. Baltimore: Johns Hopkins University Press, 2012.

Letters of Joseph J. Kinyoun. History of Medicine Division, National Library of Medicine, Bethesda, MD.

Hawgood, Barbara J. "Waldemar Mordecai Haffkine, CIE (1860–1930): prophylactic vaccination against cholera and bubonic plague in British India." *Journal of Medical Biography* 15, no. 1 (February 2007).

"Plague in Bombay–Haffkine serum." *Public Health Reports*, November 8, 1899.

"Court Asked to End the Bubonic Infamy." *San Francisco Chronicle*, May 25, 1900.

"Quarantine by the State Board." *San Francisco Call*, May 29, 1900.

CHAPTER 6: QUARANTINE

"Board of Health Confesses to Famous Expert Who Crossed the Continent at the Insistence of the New York Herald and the Call That There Is No Bubonic Plague in This City." *San Francisco Call*, May 29, 1900.

"Investigating Experts Inspect Chinatown and Fail to Find a Single Case of Any Illness." *San Francisco Call*, May 30, 1900.

"Searching for Disease in Dens of Chinatown." *San Francisco Call*, May 30, 1900.

"Sporadic Case of Bubonic Plague Discovered, but There Is Absolutely No Need for Alarm." *San Francisco Call*, May 31, 1900.

"Dr. Crowley Would Burn Down Chinatown." *San Francisco Call*, May 31, 1900.

"Danger of Plague Has Passed and Vigilance Will Insure Complete Safety of the City." *San Francisco Call*, June 1, 1900.

"Phelan in the Role of a Faker." *San Francisco Chronicle*, May 30, 1900.

"Plague Fake Put Through." *San Francisco Chronicle*, May 30, 1900.

"Plague Fake on Last Legs." *San Francisco Chronicle*, June 4, 1900.

"No State Quarantine." *San Francisco Chronicle*, June 4, 1900.

"Governor and Plague: He and Not Kinyoun Appealed to by the Government." *San Francisco Chronicle*, June 4, 1900.

"Scott Not a Subscriber." *San Francisco Chronicle*, June 5, 1900.

"He Swallowed a Thermometer." *San Francisco Chronicle*, June 3, 1900.

"Plague and the Courts." *San Francisco Chronicle*, June 5, 1900.

"Three Blows That Stagger the Board of Plague Fakers." *San Francisco Chronicle*, June 6, 1900.

"Editorial." *San Francisco Chronicle*, June 7, 1900.

"Criticism Will Cure the Trouble." *San Francisco Chronicle*, June 7, 1900.

"Inviting Counties to Act." *San Francisco Chronicle*, June 7, 1900.

"Bad Faith to the City." *San Francisco Chronicle*, June 7, 1900.

"Statements by Physicians." *San Francisco Chronicle*, June 7, 1900.

"Cases Kept Undercover." *San Francisco Chronicle*, June 10, 1900.

Letters of Joseph J. Kinyoun. History of Medicine Division, National Library of Medicine, Bethesda, MD.

"To Answer for Contempt." *San Francisco Chronicle*, June 11, 1900.

"Island Officials Puzzled." *San Francisco Chronicle*, June 13, 1900.

"Governor Officially Brands Plague Scare a Fake." *San Francisco Chronicle*, June 14, 1900.

"Plague Fake at Its End." *San Francisco Chronicle*, June 16, 1900.

CHAPTER 7: OUST THE FAKER

"Take Him Out At Once." *San Francisco Chronicle*, June 17, 1900.

"Desperate Kinyoun Commits New Outrage on San Francisco." *San Francisco Chronicle*, June 17, 1900.

"Quarantine Denounced." *San Francisco Chronicle*, June 18, 1900.

"Cited for Contempt." *San Francisco Chronicle*, June 18, 1900.

"Remove the Revengeful Man." *San Francisco Chronicle*, June 19, 1900.

"Quarantine Fake Explodes: Kinyoun Pleads for Respite." *San Francisco Chronicle*, June 19, 1900.

"His Recall Is Demanded: Angry Citizens Say That Kinyoun Must Leave." *San Francisco Chronicle*, June 20, 1900.

"Bad Faith on Kinyoun's Part." *San Francisco Chronicle*, June 22, 1900.

"Dr Kinyoun Will Answer Today." *San Francisco Chronicle*, June 26, 1900.

"Kinyoun Has Weak Defense." *San Francisco Chronicle*, June 26, 1900.

Annual Report of the Supervising Surgeon-General of the Marine-Hospital Service of the United States for the Fiscal Year 1899. Washington: Government Printing Office, 1901.

Letters of Joseph J. Kinyoun. History of Medicine Division, National Library of Medicine, Bethesda, MD.

Risse, Guenter B. *Plague, Fear, and Politics in San Francisco's Chinatown.* Baltimore: Johns Hopkins University Press, 2012.

"Has Kinyoun Gone Mad?" *San Francisco Chronicle*, October 2, 1900.

"Indecencies of Kinyoun." *San Francisco Chronicle*, October 3, 1900.

"The Doom of Kinyoun." *San Francisco Chronicle*, December 28, 1900.

CHAPTER 8: AN INFAMOUS COMPACT

"The Bubonic Plague." *Southern California Practitioner: A Monthly Journal of Medicine and Allied Science* 15, no. 7 (July 1900).

Kazanjian, Powel. "Frederick Novy and the 1901 San Francisco Plague Commission Investigation." *Clinical Infectious Diseases* 55, no. 10 (November 15, 2012).

Link, Vernon B. "A History of Plague in the United States of America." *Public Health Monograph* 26, 1955.

Kazanjian, Powel. *Frederick Novy and the Development of Bacteriology in Medicine.* New Brunswick, NJ: Rutgers University Press, 2017.

"The Governor's Message and the Plague." *Occidental Medical Times* 15, no. 2 (February 1901).

Annual Report of the Supervising Surgeon-General of the Marine-Hospital Service of the United States for the Fiscal Year 1901. Washington: Government Printing Office, 1902.

Barker, Lewellys F. "On the Clinical Aspects of Plague." *American Journal of the Medical Sciences* 122, no. 4 (October 1901).

Risse, Guenter B. *Plague, Fear, and Politics in San Francisco's Chinatown.* Baltimore: Johns Hopkins University Press, 2012.

Letters of Joseph J. Kinyoun. History of Medicine Division, National Library of Medicine, Bethesda, MD.

"The Plague, 'American Medicine,' and the 'Philadelphia Medical Journal.'" *Occidental Medical Times* 15, no. 5 (May 1901).

"Bubonic Plague." *Transactions of the Medical Society of the State of California. Thirty-First Annual Session, Sacramento, April 1901.* Vol. 31.

CHAPTER 9: AN IMPOSSIBLE TASK

Risse, Guenter B. *Plague, Fear, and Politics in San Francisco's Chinatown.* Baltimore: Johns Hopkins University Press, 2012.

Annual Report of the Supervising Surgeon-General of the Marine-Hospital Service of the United States for the Fiscal Year 1901. Washington: Government Printing Office, 1902.

Letters of Rupert Lee Blue. Unpublished. Collection of J. Michael Hughes.

Chase, Marilyn. *The Barbary Plague.* New York: Random House, 2003.

Flexure, Abraham. "Medical Education in America." *Atlantic,* June 1910.

Weissman, Gerald. "Rats, Lice, and Zinsser." *Emerging Infectious Diseases* 11, no. 3 (March 2005).

Zinsser, Hans. *Rats, Lice and History.* New York: Transaction, 2017.

Larson, Erik. *Isaac's Storm.* New York: Random House, 1999.

Medical Sentinel 7, no. 1 (January 1899).

"Mrs. Rupert Blue, the Guest." *San Francisco Call,* May 24, 1901.

Sharp, Sally. "About Pretty Miss Mary Barber: Some Prominent Society Swells." *San Francisco Call*, May 26, 1901.

"Santiago Hero on the Sumner: Lieutenant Victor Blue Home from Manila on Leave." *San Francisco Call*, August 19, 1901.

"Thirty Four Perished in Montana Train Wreck." *San Francisco Chronicle*, September 1, 1901.

CHAPTER 10: A MOST PECULIAR TEAM

Annual Report of the Supervising Surgeon-General of the Marine-Hospital Service of the United States for the Fiscal Year 1901. Washington: Government Printing Office, 1902.

Chase, Marilyn. *The Barbary Plague*. New York: Random House, 2003.

Risse, Guenter B. *Plague, Fear, and Politics in San Francisco's Chinatown*. Baltimore: Johns Hopkins University Press, 2012.

Sullivan, Robert. *Rats: Observations on the History and Habitat of the City's Most Unwanted Inhabitants*. New York: Bloomsbury, 2004.

Berth, John. *The Black Death: The Great Mortality of 1348–1350, A Brief History with Documents*. New York: Palgrave Macmillan, 2005.

Warlock, Nukhet. *Plague and Empire in the Early Modern Mediterranean World*. New York: Cambridge University Press, 2015.

"Plague and Fleas." *Nature*, November 21, 1907.

Cohn, Samuel K. "Epidemiology of the Black Death and Successive Waves of Plague." *Medical History Supplement* 27 (2008).

Bray, R. S. *Armies of Pestilence: The Impact of Disease on History*. Cambridge: James Clarke & Co., 1996.

Simon, M., M. L. Goldey, and P. D. Mouriquand. "Paul-Louis Simond and His Discovery of Plague Transmission by Rat Fleas: a Centenary." *Journal of the Royal Society of Medicine* 91, no. 2 (February 1998).

Gross, Ludwik. "How the Plague Bacillus and Its Transmutation Through Fleas Were Discovered: Reminiscences from My Years at the Pasteur Institute in Paris." *Current Science* 70, no. 12 (June 25, 1996).

Petrie, G. F. "Rats and Plague." *Scientific American*, February 11, 1911.

Wyman, Walter. *The Bubonic Plague*. Washington: Government Printing Office, 1900.

Letters of Rupert Lee Blue. Unpublished. Collection of J. Michael Hughes.

"The Bubonic Plague Fake." *San Francisco Chronicle*, October 21, 1901.

"Warns against Apathy on Chinese Exclusion." *San Francisco Chronicle*, November 18, 1901.

"More about the Plague Fake." *San Francisco Chronicle*, November 28, 1901.

"The Chinese in Chinatown." *San Francisco Chronicle*, February 20, 1902.

CHAPTER 11: AS SOON AS POSSIBLE

"Dr. Blue's Wife Secures Divorce." *San Francisco Chronicle*, April 17, 1902.

Douglas, Lawrence, and Taylor Hansen. "The Chinese Six Companies of San Francisco and the Smuggling of Chinese Immigrants Across the U.S.-Mexico Border, 1882–1930." *Journal of the Southwest* 48, no. 1 (Spring 2006).

Annual Report of the Supervising Surgeon-General of the Marine-Hospital Service of the United States for the Fiscal Year 1901. Washington: Government Printing Office, 1902.

Risse, Guenter B. *Plague, Fear, and Politics in San Francisco's Chinatown.* Baltimore: Johns Hopkins University Press, 2012.

"Suggestions for City Improvement: Why Chinatown Has Remained Where It Is." *San Francisco News Letter*, April 30, 1902. Accessed via the Virtual Museum of San Francisco at http://www.sfmuseum.net/hist9/chinatown.html.

Chase, Marilyn. *The Barbary Plague.* New York: Random House, 2003.

CHAPTER 12: THE UNPLEASANT PAST

Letters of Rupert Lee Blue. Unpublished. Collection of J. Michael Hughes.

"A Plea for the Slumless City." *Our Day*, January 1906.

"The Public Health." *The Medical Times: A Monthly Journal of Medicine, Surgery and the Collateral Sciences* 33 (January–December 1905).

Chase, Marilyn. *The Barbary Plague.* New York: Random House, 2003.

Annual Report of the Supervising Surgeon-General of the Marine-Hospital Service of the United States for the Fiscal Year 1902. Washington: Government Printing Office, 1903.

Risse, Guenter B. *Plague, Fear, and Politics in San Francisco's Chinatown.* Baltimore: Johns Hopkins University Press, 2012.

Annual Report of the Supervising Surgeon-General of the Marine-Hospital Service of the United States for the Fiscal Year 1905. Washington: Government Printing Office, 1906.

CHAPTER 13: FOR GOD'S SAKE, SEND FOOD

"Enrico Caruso and the 1906 Earthquake." *The Theatre* 6, no. 65 (July 1, 1906). Accessed via the Virtual Museum of the City of San Francisco at http://www.sfmuseum.net/1906/ew19.html.

"Jack London and the Great Earthquake and Fire." Accessed via the Virtual Museum of the City of San Francisco at http://www.sfmuseum.net/hist5/jlondon.html.

Hansen, Gladys. "A Great Civic Drama." Accessed via the Virtual Museum of the City of San Francisco at http://www.sfmuseum.net/hist/timeline.html.

Annual Report of the Director of the Mint to the Secretary of the Treasury Fiscal Year Ended June 30, 1906. Washington: Government Printing Office, 1906. Accessed at https://www.usmint.gov/learn/history/historical-documents/san-francisco-great-earthquake-and-fire.

Miller, Joaquin. "A Fire So Richly Fed." *Oakland Tribune*, May 6, 1906. Accessed via the Virtual Museum of the City of San Francisco at http://www.sfmuseum .net/1906/ew5.html.

"Little Light for Weeks to Come." *San Francisco Chronicle*, April 30, 1906.

Freeman, Frederick (Lt.). "Navy Firefighting Operations." April 30, 1906. Accessed via the Virtual Museum of the City of San Francisco at http://www.sfmuseum .net/1906/usn.html.

"Thomas Chase's Eyewitness Account at the Ferry Building." Accessed via the Virtual Museum of the City of San Francisco at http://www.sfmuseum.net/1906/ ew1.html.

Public Health Reports 21, Part 1, May 11, 1906.

George Torney, telegram to the Surgeon General of the U.S. Army, April 20, 1906. Accessed from the National Archives at https://www.archives.gov/exhibits/ sf-earthquake-and-fire/rebirth.html.

Winchester, Simon. *A Crack in the Edge of the World: America and the Great California Earthquake of 1906.* New York: Harper Perennial, 2005.

"Mr. Bacigalupi's Own Story." *Edison Phonograph Monthly*, May 1906. Accessed via the Virtual Museum of the City of San Francisco at http://www.sfmuseum .org/1906/ew16.html.

"The 1906 Earthquake: Eyewitness Accounts." *100 Years after the San Francisco Quake.* NPR, April 11, 2006. Accessed at https://www.npr.org/templates/ story/story.php?storyId=5334623.

Letters of Rupert Lee Blue. Unpublished. Collection of J. Michael Hughes.

Risse, Guenter B. *Plague, Fear, and Politics in San Francisco's Chinatown.* Baltimore: Johns Hopkins University Press, 2012.

Chase, Marilyn. *The Barbary Plague.* New York: Random House, 2003.

CHAPTER 14: TWO PERCENT

"When You Go to San Francisco Seek to Relieve Suffering." *Organized Labor*, May 5, 1906. Accessed via the Virtual Museum of the City of San Francisco at http://www.sfmuseum.net/press/clips19.html.

"Rebuilding San Francisco Following the 1906 Earthquake." Accessed via the Virtual Museum of the City of San Francisco at http://www.sfmuseum.org/1906/ rebuild.html.

"Mayor Schmitz Bans Coolie Labor for Reconstruction." Accessed via the Virtual Museum of the City of San Francisco at http://www.sfmuseum.net/1906.2/ asiatic.html.

Chase, Marilyn. *The Barbary Plague*. New York: Random House, 2003.

Rucker, William Colby. "The Relation of the California Ground Squirrel (*Citellus Beechyi*) to Bubonic Plague." *Bulletin of the Wisconsin Natural History Society* 8, no. 3 (July 1910).

"The Ravages of Rats." *San Francisco Chronicle*, June 14, 1907.

"Authorities Make Report on the Bubonic Plague." *San Francisco Chronicle*, August 16, 1907.

"Closing Out Relief Work." *San Francisco Chronicle*, August 20, 1907.

"Editorial." *Pacific Medical Journal* 50, no. 10 (October 1907).

"Scout the Idea of an Epidemic." *San Francisco Chronicle*, September 14, 1907.

"Small Danger from Alleged Plague." *San Francisco Chronicle*, September 21, 1907.

Eradicating Plague from San Francisco. San Francisco Citizen's Health Committee Report. 1909.

Blue, Rupert. "Anti-Plague Measures in San Francisco, California, U.S.A." *Journal of Hygiene* 11, no. 1 (1909).

Blue, Rupert. "The Underlying Principles of Anti-Plague Measures." *California State Journal of Medicine* 6, no. 8 (August 1908).

Strother, E. French. "How the Plague Was Driven Out." *California Weekly*, April 9, 1909.

"How to Catch Rats." *Marin Journal*, March 12, 1908.

Ziv, Stav. "Chronicle Founder Shot Dead in Feud, 1880." *San Francisco Chronicle*, April 9, 2012.

Reno, Nilda. "Days Gone By: San Francisco Newspaper History Riddled with Bullets." *Mercury News*, October 4, 2010.

Kennedy, Robert C. "On This Day: November 10, 1906." *New York Times*. Accessed at http://www.nytimes.com/learning/general/onthisday/harp/1110.html.

Rucker, William Colby. " 'Frisco's Fight with Bubonic Plague." *Technical World*, November 1909.

CHAPTER 15: THE WORST CORNER OF HELL

Chase, Marilyn. *The Barbary Plague*. New York: Random House, 2003.

"Officials Will Confer." *San Francisco Chronicle*, November 7, 1907.

"Finds but Two Alleged Cases." *San Francisco Chronicle*, February 22, 1908.

Letters of Rupert Lee Blue. Unpublished. Collection of J. Michael Hughes.

Eradicating Plague from San Francisco. San Francisco Citizen's Health Committee Report. 1909.

"Citizens Urged to War on Rats." *San Francisco Call*, January 29, 1908.

"Club Women to Fight the Rats." *San Francisco Chronicle*, February 8, 1908.

"Slaughter of Rats Planned." *San Francisco Chronicle*, February 12, 1908.

"Street Banquet is Given by Merchants." *San Francisco Chronicle*, March 22, 1907.

"Mayor and Party to Visit City Wards." *San Francisco Chronicle*, March 26, 1907.

"Public Health up to People." *San Francisco Call*, February 8, 1908.

"Greatest Naval Parade Planned." *San Francisco Chronicle*, April 7, 1908.

"Fleet Visitors to Throng City." *San Francisco Chronicle*, April 10, 1908.

"Plans for the Reception of the Fleet." *San Francisco Chronicle*, May 3, 1908.

"Shoots Himself When Grief Is Unbearable." *San Francisco Chronicle*, April 17, 1908.

CHAPTER 16: ONE OF CALIFORNIA'S ADOPTED SONS

"The Most Powerful Naval Force Ever Assembled in the Pacific." *San Francisco Chronicle*, May 3, 1908.

"Warm Greeting of 'God's Own Land.'" *San Francisco Chronicle*, May 7, 1908.

"First Vision of the Atlantic Fleet." *San Francisco Chronicle*. May 7, 1908.

"How the Fleet Fared in Frisco." *Pacific Commercial Advertiser*, May 30, 1908.

Nolte, Carl. "Great White Fleet Visited San Francisco 100 Years Ago." *San Francisco Chronicle*, May 6, 2008.

Chase, Marilyn. *The Barbary Plague*. New York: Random House, 2003.

Fox, Carroll. "Identification of Fleas at San Francisco, Cal." *Public Health Reports*, September 25, 1908.

Strickland, C. "The Biology of Ceratophyllus fasciatus Bosc, the Common Rat-Flea of Great Britain." *Journal of Hygiene* 14, no. 2 (July 1914).

Simpson, W. J. "The Croonian Lectures on Plague, Delivered before the Royal College of Physicians on June 18, 20, 25, and 27." *Journal of Tropical Medicine and Hygiene* 10, no. 14 (July 15, 1907).

Letters of Rupert Lee Blue. Unpublished. Collection of J. Michael Hughes.

Eradicating Plague from San Francisco. San Francisco Citizen's Health Committee Report. 1909.

"Brilliant Banquet in Dr. Blue's Honor." *San Francisco Call*, April 1, 1909.

Rucker, William Colby. "The Relation of the California Ground Squirrel (*Citellus Beechyi*) to Bubonic Plague." *Bulletin of the Wisconsin Natural History Society* 8, no. 3 (July 1910).

CHAPTER 17: CAST ASIDE

"Plague-Prevention Work." *Public Health Reports* 26, no. 34 (August 25, 1911).

Blue, Rupert. "Squirrel Eradication." *Proceedings of the Fifty-Eighth Fruit Growers' Convention of the State of California*. Sacramento: W. W. Shannon, 1911.

Chase, Marilyn. *The Barbary Plague*. New York: Random House, 2003.

Letters of Rupert Lee Blue. Unpublished. Collection of J. Michael Hughes.

"Dr. Blue Assured of Wyman's Job." *San Francisco Call*, January 5, 1912.

"Bubonic Plague Still a Menace." *New York Times*, April 23, 1910.

"Physicians Approve New Code of Ethics." *New York Times*, June 6, 1912.

"Many Savants Join in Hygiene Congress." *New York Times*, September 21, 1912.

"Miracles of Modern Sanitary Science for All to See." *New York Times*, September 8, 1912.

"Fighting against Plague." *New York Times*, June 30, 1914.

"Blue Heads Plague War." *New York Times*, July 4, 1914.

"Rat-Proofing American Cities." *New York Times*, July 25, 1915.

"Medical Men Face Needs of War." *New York Times*, June 5, 1917.

"31 New Influenza Cases in New York." *New York Times*, September 21, 1918.

Stobbe, Mike. *Surgeon General's Warning: How Politics Crippled the Nation's Doctors.* Oakland, CA: University of California Press, 2014.

Morabia, Alfredo. "Joseph Goldberger's Research on the Prevention of Pellagra." *Journal of the Royal Society of Medicine* 101, no. 11 (November 1, 2008).

"Bubonic Plague in New Orleans." *California State Journal of Medicine* 12, no. 10 (October 1914).

Campanella, Richard. "The Battle against Bubonic Plague; 100 Years Ago, New Orleans Waged War on Rats." *New Orleans Times-Picayune*, August 5, 2014.

"Plague-Eradicative Work." *Public Health Reports*, December 25, 1914.

Duffy, John. *The Sanitarians: A History of American Public Health.* Urbana: University of Illinois Press, 1992.

Barry, John M. "How the Horrific 1918 Flu Spread across America." *Smithsonian*, November 2017.

Barry, John M. *The Great Influenza: The Story of the Deadliest Pandemic in History.* New York: Viking Penguin, 2004.

CHAPTER 18: A HERO ONCE MORE

Deverell, William. *Whitewashed Adobe: The Rise of Los Angeles and the Remaking of Its Mexican Past.* Berkeley: University of California Press, 2004.

Matsumoto, Valerie J., and Blake Allmendinger. *Over the Edge: Remapping the American West.* Berkeley: University of California Press, 1999.

"No Spread of Disease." *Los Angeles Times*, November 7, 1924.

"No New Pneumonic Cases." *Los Angeles Times*, November 8, 1924.

Molina, Natalia. *Fit to Be Citizens? Public Health and Race in Los Angeles, 1879–1939.* Berkeley: University of California Press, 2006.

"No New Plague Cases Show Up." *Los Angeles Times*, November 9, 1924.

"End Seen in Pneumonic Outbreaks." *Los Angeles Times*, November 10, 1924.

"Quarantine for Plague Area Lifted." *Los Angeles Times*, November 14, 1924.

"Little Mexico Honors Its Heroine." *Los Angeles Times*, November 14, 1924.

"Governor Gratified at End of Plague Menace." *Los Angeles Times*, November 16, 1924.

"Rat Clean-up in City Urged." *Los Angeles Times*, November 19, 1924.

"Go On with the Rat Killing." *Los Angeles Times*, November 22, 1924.

"War Declared against Rats." *Los Angeles Times*, November 22, 1924.

"Advertising Tour Planned." *Los Angeles Times*, November 27, 1924.

"Rat War Death Toll Is Heavy." *Los Angeles Times*, November 30, 1924.

"Early Shopping Food Pages." *Los Angeles Times*, May 12, 1925.

"Plan to Ban Rats Lauded." *Los Angeles Times*, November 25, 1925.

Davis, Mike. *Ecology of Fear: Los Angeles and the Imagination of Disaster*. New York: Vintage, 1999.

Rasmussen, Cecilia. "In 1924 Los Angeles, a Scourge from the Middle Ages." *Los Angeles Times*, March 5, 2006.

Annual Report of the Surgeon General of the Public Health Service of the United States for the Fiscal Year 1925. Washington: Government Printing Office, 1926.

INDEX

BLACK DEATH AT THE GOLDEN GATE

David K. Randall

BLACK DEATH AT THE GOLDEN GATE

David K. Randall

DISCUSSION QUESTIONS

1. David K. Randall talks about how Polish women armed with base-ball bats and butcher knives patrolled the streets ready to combat health inspectors during the smallpox epidemic of 1894 (p. 5). Even after one confirmed death by the bubonic plague, the *San Francisco Chronicle* and other city newspapers called the scare "nothing but a ploy by the Board of Health to receive more fund-ing" (p. 46). Why was fear and distrust for public health officials so widespread? Does this change as the book progresses? What is different today?

2. Even though San Francisco was festering with health issues and the population doubled between 1870 and 1885, Randall says that spending on sanitation, hospitals, and other forms of medical care and prevention fell by 20 percent. Why would the city believe "it was a waste of money at best and a swindle at worst" (p. 35), even as public health was failing?

3. Randall discusses misguided notions about the plague, such as that it "could only flourish in hot climates, and even then only among those who ate rice instead of a more muscular European diet cen-tered on meat" (p. 46). What are the roots, and the consequences, of this belief?

4. Governor Henry Gage was insistent in denying the outbreak. What were his motivations for denying the existence of the plague even as the death toll continued to rise?

5. Randall states that "the only thing uniting the Chinese tongs and the white men in power was their willingness to do anything to suppress the truth of plague in the district" (p. 147). Why did the

Chinese Six Companies want to suppress the truth about the outbreak?

6. How was Rupert Blue able to succeed where Joseph Kinyoun failed?

7. Did any of the elements of this narrative strike you as similar to the present day? What can we learn from the way the plague was, and was not, kept at bay?

*Available only on the Norton website